Eating to Learn, Learning to Eat

Critical Issues in Health and Medicine

Edited by Rima D. Apple, University of Wisconsin–Madison,
and Janet Golden, Rutgers University, Camden

Growing criticism of the U.S. healthcare system is coming from consumers, politicians, the media, activists, and healthcare professionals. Critical Issues in Health and Medicine is a collection of books that explores these contemporary dilemmas from a variety of perspectives, among them political, legal, historical, sociological, and comparative, and with attention to crucial dimensions such as race, gender, ethnicity, sexuality, and culture.

Eating to Learn, Learning to Eat

The Origins of School Lunch in the United States

A. R. Ruis

Rutgers University Press

New Brunswick, Camden, and Newark, New Jersey, and London

Library of Congress Cataloging-in-Publication Data

Names: Ruis, A. R., 1979– author.
Title: Eating to learn, learning to eat : the origins of school lunch in the United
    States / A.R. Ruis.
Description: New Brunswick : Rutgers University Press, [2017] | Series: Critical
    issues in health and medicine | Includes bibliographical references and index.
Identifiers: LCCN 2016043281| ISBN 9780813590486 (hardcover : alk. paper) |
    ISBN 9780813584072 (pbk. : alk. paper) | ISBN 9780813584089 (e-book (epub)) |
    ISBN 9780813584096 (e-book (web pdf)) | ISBN 9780813590868 (e-book (mobi))
Subjects: LCSH: National school lunch program—History.
Classification: LCC LB3479.U6 R85 2017 | DDC 371.7/160973—dc23
LC record available at https://lccn.loc.gov/2016043281

A British Cataloging-in-Publication record for this book is available from the
British Library.

♾ The paper used in this publication meets the requirements of the American
National Standard for Information Sciences—Permanence of Paper for Printed
Library Materials, ANSI Z39.48–1992.

www.rutgersuniversitypress.org

Manufactured in the United States of America

For JWL, RDA, NMR, SPR, and TMP, whose full identities I leave as an exercise for the reader

Contents

Abbreviations

AICP   Association for Improving the Condition of the Poor
(New York City)

CSEC   Chicago School Extension Committee

NSLP   National School Lunch Program

PTA   Parent-Teacher Association

SLC   School Lunch Committee (New York City)

SLIC   School Lunch Inquiry Committee (New York City)

SMA   Surplus Marketing Administration

USDA   United States Department of Agriculture

WPA   Works Progress Administration/Work Projects
Administration

Abbreviations

Eating to Learn, Learning to Eat

Introduction

The penny lunch has spread faster than the measles. There seems
no immunity for it. Everybody is taking it.
—J. M. Withrow, Cincinnati Board of Education (1933)[1]

If it is true that everyone has a story about food, then everyone probably has a horror story about school lunches. When the pseudony-
mous teacher Mrs. Q began eating federally subsidized lunches with
her students in 2010, documenting each meal on her blog, she was
often appalled by the quality of the food. Lunches were something to
be "survived" rather than enjoyed. "The patty was how do you say
nothing like any hamburger I have ever eaten. Mystery meat in every
sense," she wrote of her meal on 12 January. "I also really wanted more
than just six tator tots. The fruit cup was NOT FROZEN, so I ate it."
On 15 December, near the end of her experiment, she revealed how
difficult her one-year commitment to eating school lunches had been.
"I feel like I'm breaking out of prison on Friday. Having to eat school
lunch has almost been harder psychologically than physically though
it has been tough in every way." With just twenty minutes for lunch,
including time spent getting to and from the cafeteria and waiting in
line for food, the children at her school seem more like the victims of a

ruthless utilitarianism than the beneficiaries of a once-beloved federal health and welfare program.[2]

While Mrs. Q was enduring school lunches with her students, a reform coalition was developing around childhood obesity, inactivity, and nutritional health. Nearly a third of the nation's young were overweight or obese, a substantial increase in prevalence since the 1970s. According to the U.S. Department of Defense, 75 percent of Americans seventeen to twenty-four years of age were ineligible to serve in the armed forces, and overweight/obesity was the leading cause of rejection on medical grounds.[3] On the premise that children's poor nutrition and lack of physical fitness threatened public health and national security, a number of new health initiatives were launched in 2010, including First Lady Michelle Obama's Let's Move! and Mission: Readiness, a coalition backed by a group of retired military leaders. They joined an already large and growing faction of education and public health organizations promoting increased federal funding and higher nutrition standards for school meals; the removal of junk foods, candy, and sodas from school grounds; and the expansion of public health nutrition and physical education in schools.

The combination of increased public attention to school meals and mounting political pressure for major revisions to national nutrition policy ultimately secured legislative action. By the end of the year, President Barack Obama had signed into law the Healthy, Hunger-Free Kids Act. The act substantially reformed the National School Lunch Program (NSLP), the longest-running children's health and welfare program in U.S. history and a cornerstone of the nation's public health nutrition and food security infrastructure. Among other changes, the act increased federal reimbursement rates for school meals by six cents per meal (in 2010, the federal reimbursement rates were $2.72 for each free lunch and $2.32 for each reduced-price lunch[4]); it authorized schools to provide free meals to all students based on community eligibility if at least 40 percent of attending students would qualify for free meals individually; it required periodic audits of the nutritional content of the meals served in schools; and it stipulated that participating schools must establish a "wellness policy," "including, at a minimum, goals for nutrition promotion and education, physical activity, and other school-based activities that promote student wellness." Furthermore, it required all foods not included in the federally subsidized meals but sold on school grounds, including snacks and beverages dispensed from vending machines, to conform to nutrition standards established by the U.S. Department of Agriculture.[5]

The movement for reformed nutrition policy, which culminated in the Healthy, Hunger-Free Kids Act, united a range of stakeholders—food processors and distributors, health professionals, education and community leaders, school foodservice associations—and received limited bipartisan support in Congress at a time when cooperation between Democrats and Republicans was particularly rare. Improving school meals, and through them the nutritional health of children, seemed to be an issue that most could support. But by 2012, as the new requirements came into effect, they sparked perhaps the most extensive and divisive political battle over school meals since the NSLP began in 1947.[6]

Established by the National School Lunch Act of 1946, today the NSLP operates in more than 100,000 schools and childcare centers in the United States and provides free or low-cost meals to more than 31 million children every school day.[7] Students consume as many as half of their meals at school, and each school meal may represent more than half of a student's daily caloric intake.[8] For seventy years, however, schools participating in the NSLP have struggled to provide appetizing, nutritious, low-cost meals that satisfy both federal requirements and children's tastes. Expected to address health and welfare concerns ranging from poverty and hunger to malnutrition and childhood obesity, saddled with incentives to rely heavily on processed foods and surplus commodities, increasingly dependent on private food and management companies, and chronically underfunded, the NSLP—despite its many successes—came to symbolize the failures of American nutrition policy. But while there has long been concern that the NSLP is "deeply flawed," the historian Susan Levine has argued, Americans have remained "intensely committed to the idea of a school lunch program, particularly one that offers free meals to poor children."[9]

That commitment, as this book shows, long predates the NSLP itself. Although most historical work has focused on the NSLP,[10] the national program was established only after decades of experimentation and development at the local level. Before 1900, only a few day schools were experimenting with systems to provide food for students; in general, the care and feeding of children were regarded as the responsibility of the home, beyond the purview of public education. By 1913, however, at least forty-six cities across the United States had regular meal programs in at least some schools.[11] Numerous cities, as well as many one-room and consolidated rural schools, were implementing meal services for students by the 1920s. According to one 1924 study, of the 286 U.S. cities with populations of more than 25,000 people, at least 134 (47 percent) had some kind of lunch program.[12] In the 1923–1924 school year, rural schools served 1.8 million hot meals, and urban schools served 2.7 million; the programs grossed over $1 million a day in sales, and many served free or reduced-price meals.[13] By the time Congress passed the National School Lunch Act in 1946, upward of 8 million children at 60,000 schools were already participating in some kind of school lunch or milk program.[14] Although the development of school meal programs was not uniform in all areas, feeding children in schools ultimately became the primary public health nutrition initiative for children in the United States.

The history of school meals suggests that education and health authorities have struggled for more than a hundred years to establish programs that address hunger and malnourishment, promote nutritional health, and satisfy children's appetites while keeping costs low and maintaining political support. While some of the difficulties are practical or logistical, others involve fundamental conflicts over the extent to which nutritional health intervention should be undertaken and the best ways to do so. Health experts and nutritionists disagree, for example, about the relative importance of altering individual behavior and fostering universal, structural changes. Is it better to limit children's choices so that they must consume nutritious foods, or teach them to select a healthful meal from a wide range of options, as they must do outside of school? To what extent should the school lunch balance nutritive considerations with children's tastes and preferences? Should reforms be directed at individual consumers, such as the children themselves, or at food systems, such as the ecologies of production, processing, distribution, and consumption?[15]

These questions, which must be addressed in a complex and constantly changing political landscape, reflect the constant negotiation of responsibility for children's nutritional health and the tension between individual choice and communal benefit.

This book does not offer specific solutions to these problems, but rather explores how and why school meal programs came to have the form ultimately codified by the National School Lunch Act. While the NSLP was in part a response to specific concerns about children's access to sufficient and sufficiently nourishing food during the Great Depression and World War II, many of the issues that shaped school meal policies and practices arose decades earlier. Exploring the local origins of school meals shows that early programs were far more varied—and in some cases, far more successful—than those of the consolidated federal system. Local programs responded to local issues, but they also faced different pressures. Because the federal government had little involvement in public health or education prior to the New Deal, the politics of school meals reflected state and municipal differences in law, policy, and social context. Those differences can be seen in the different patterns of development that characterized early school meal programs, but they also reveal the underlying debates that shaped the evolution of national school meal policy.

Though recent debates over school meals are different from those of the past, they are nonetheless shaped by historical context. Because nutrition and health are defined by sociopolitical negotiations as much as by biomedical expertise, historical perspective is critical to a complete understanding of the bases on which national nutrition policy has been constructed. By exploring the origins of school meal initiatives, this book endeavors to explain why it was (and to some extent, has continued to be) so difficult to establish meal programs that satisfy the often competing interests of children, schools, health authorities, politicians, and the food industry, which itself includes producers, processors, distributors, and others who play a significant role in the country's food system. Indeed, Americans are once again debating the affordances and limitations of school meals, and as in the past, a key issue is the lack of clear data on the actual costs and benefits of feeding children in schools.

Perusal of major U.S. news sources after 2010 reveals a concerted and increasingly contentious public and professional discussion of school meals: about the role of school meals in the reduction of hunger and malnourishment; about the relative benefits of home-packed versus school meals; about schoolchildren's generally poor dietary choices and nutritional health; about the labor force that has been reduced to reheating pre-prepared meals; about the quality and impact of school meal nutrition standards and other federal requirements; about the quality of the food served; about how much of the food served in school meals children actually eat; and about numerous ways that school meals could be improved nutritionally, logistically, environmentally, and gastronomically. Indeed, similar discussions were common over a century ago, when meal programs were first established at schools across the country. This contiguity of discourse across more than a century reflects the fundamentally social process through which understanding of nutrition is constructed. Which foods are healthful (or not), what constitutes a meal, how foods should be prepared and consumed, and even what counts as "food" are not empirical questions to be answered in labs or clinics but social questions continually addressed through the combination of scientific, cultural, and political—but also historical—processes.

This book examines the nature of these processes in the creation of school meal programs, first at the local and then at the national level, in the decades leading up to the passage of the National School Lunch Act.[16] Chapter 1 explores how social changes beginning in the late nineteenth century—urbanization, industrialization, opposition to child labor, and compulsory education laws—drew attention to children's poor nutritional health. As more and more children attended school, for more hours in the day and more days in the year, the school became a central civic institution and a site for unprecedented state intervention in the lives of children. Once charged with instilling basic competencies such as the three Rs (reading, 'riting, and 'rithmetic), by the early twentieth century urban schools were providing numerous services besides classroom education, including medical inspection, nursing, eye and dental care, physical education and recreational activities, special classes for disabled students, and ultimately meals.

The school became the primary locus for children's health work due to its extensive contact with children and their families, its integration into state and local bureaucracies, and its stabile infrastructure. With more parents working outside the home and children spending more time in class, the school also became the primary site for the negotiation between home and state of responsibility for children's health and welfare. School meals, as they were realized in different contexts, reflected the extent to which the state began to provide not only for children's educations but also for their care.

To explore these processes in more detail, chapters 2 and 3 provide detailed case studies of the establishment of school meal programs in Chicago and New York City, respectively. These were the two largest cities in the nation, with the two largest public school systems. In many ways, they were quite similar: both were densely populated cities with enormous economies, machine politics, widespread poverty, and antiquated schools ill equipped to deal with either the sheer number of children or their ethnic and linguistic diversity. Despite what in many ways were similar circumstances, the development of school meal programs in the two cities was markedly different.

The Chicago Board of Education not only supported efforts to establish school meal programs but often lobbied for them. In large part due to this advocacy, Chicago soon developed the most extensive school meal program in the country. The board's efforts, however, were limited by perceived legal restrictions on educational spending and middle-class fears of socialism and undeserved charity. To avert these problems, the board partnered with the women's clubs of Chicago and ran the school meal program largely at cost, using receipts from the sale of food to cover major expenses. Although reliance on sales circumvented legal restrictions and made it possible to serve meals in more schools, it also privileged popular foods over nutritious ones and fiscal parsimony over health promotion.

In New York City, the Board of Education wanted little to do with school meals, but it granted permission to a private charity composed of home economists, physicians, and philanthropists to serve meals in schools provided the city incurred no costs. Just ten years later, the organization was serving complete, nutritious meals in almost 20 percent of the city's schools, even planning menus in accordance with different ethnic tastes and religious restrictions. Although the group hoped to transfer control of the pilot program to the Board of Education, where it could enjoy more stable funding and develop into a city-wide initiative, the board abdicated responsibility. Only after sustained pressure from concerned citizens, medical organizations—including the Board of Health—and the Board of Aldermen did the Board of Education finally accept responsibility for the program. However, apathy and political corruption had caused the initiative to stagnate under Board of Education oversight, and many of the city's schools lost their meal services or saw them replaced with profit-driven concessionaires. Not until the 1930s did the city manage, with state and federal assistance, to restore the school meal program to its former level of operation.

Each of these two case studies highlights a central challenge that early school meal advocates faced. The case of Chicago illustrates the legal issues that influenced development of publicly funded foodservice. Most states granted relatively broad powers to school boards, but spending state money to feed children fell into something of a legal gray area. Barring legislative action to specifically authorize the expenditure of public funds for free or reduced-price meals, which most states did not undertake, it was left to the school boards and the courts to decide just how flexible each state's public education charter was. The case of New York City illustrates the sociopolitical issues that influenced development of publicly funded school meal programs. Although a private, voluntary organization demonstrated that the city could serve warm, nutritious, ethnically preferable meals at scale and at minimal expense, civic authorities and community leaders were divided on the importance of doing so as a service of the school. These divisions reflected disagreement not only over the role of the school but also over the place of the state in ensuring the health of children. In exploring these issues, this chapter also examines how diverse networks of public and private interests with a stake in school meal programs formed to advance different agendas.

While school meal programs began in the cities, it was not long before rural schools began to feed children as well. Chapter 4 examines the origins of these programs, focusing on the upper Midwest. Because of significantly lower tax revenues and highly decentralized schooling, community involvement and technical ingenuity were critical in rural areas. Most rural schools had minuscule budgets, no labor source beyond teachers and students, no cooking or food preparation facilities beyond a wood-burning stove, and they often lacked even a source of fresh water. Long neglected by public health professionals—due in part to the low population densities and in part to the supposedly intrinsic healthfulness of the country—rural areas, for the first time in U.S. history, had become less healthy than urban regions by the turn of the twentieth century. This prompted an expansion of state and county health infrastructure and brought health experts to regions previously unserved. In particular, home economists, state extension agents, and public health nurses taught classes on nutrition and hygiene and helped rural schools develop lunch programs that required minimal equipment, preparation, and funding.

Rural school meal programs were not as comprehensive as those developed in cities—at best, most one-room schools could provide little more than a warm dish or simple side, such as hot cocoa or baked potato—but it took remarkable ingenuity to accomplish even that feat with extremely limited resources. By finding creative and inexpensive solutions to the problems faced by rural schools, many states significantly expanded meal programs through the efforts of extension services, state and county health departments, and county normal schools.

Chapters 5 and 6 explore the entry of the federal government into nutrition work, first as a part of New Deal food relief efforts, and then in the attempt to legislate permanent federal support for school meal programs. The investment of federal dollars into programs that had previously relied mostly on local funding affected both policy and implementation. During the 1930s, school meals remained a key means of addressing hunger and malnutrition among children, but they also became the basis of a demand-side solution to the "farm problem," the sluggish development—and often outright instability—of the country's agricultural economy. Federal school meal initiatives, and ultimately the NSLP, attempted to merge food security and agricultural protection with hunger alleviation and malnutrition prevention. In principle, it was a "two birds, one stone" solution; in practice, the NSLP privileged the interests of producers over those of consumers, and school meals became more an outlet for surplus foods than a fully realized nutrition health program for children.

The NSLP was a political triumph, but in many respects a public health failure. On one hand, reformers secured a permanent, publicly funded foundation for school meal programs, making the provision of food an integral part of the school health program. Never before had the federal government become directly involved in the conduct of schooling, and the NSLP soon became the nation's most extensive national health and welfare program for school-aged children. On the other hand, the NSLP had virtually none of the features that reformers had long worked to make central to school meal programs. It contained no universal free meals, no educational component, no protections against discrimination, structural or individual, only the most minimal nutrition standards, no specific health agenda, and no provision for training or supervision. Health and education authorities had envisioned a national program in which children would eat to learn but also learn to eat, yet they managed to secure only the former.

Chapter 1

"The Old-Fashioned Lunch Box . . . Seems Likely to Be Extinct"

The Promise of School Meals in the United States

"I grant that our school children have food enough and, in the main, good food," Horace Makechnie declared at the 1897 meeting of the American Medical Association, "but are they nourished?" Invoking a rhetorical device that would become a cliché in subsequent years— "What! starvation around tables loaded with food?"—Makechnie called attention to one of the many child health concerns that arose in the wake of compulsory schooling. With more and more American children spending long hours away from home, he warned, "we cannot afford to systematically starve our children even by an indirect way, even in a mild degree."[1]

Makechnie was not the first to express concern over the effects of schools and schooling on children's health; from the time of Horace Mann, physicians had written about the potential health consequences of poorly constructed school buildings and insalubrious educational practices. But with the expansion of compulsory education laws, the majority of which were enacted in the late nineteenth and early twentieth centuries, came a new health policy issue: If state-mandated attendance at school caused or exacerbated child health problems, to what extent was the state responsible for addressing those problems?

By removing young children from their homes for the purpose of educating them, the state implicitly assumed responsibility for their well-being. However, the extent to which that responsibility included feeding children was—and has remained to the present day—a socially and politically contentious issue. Few things were so closely associated with private, household affairs as the care and feeding of children. To make children's diets a public concern, even in part, challenged deep-seated beliefs about the balance between private and public responsibilities, the proper functions of the public school, and the role of the state in children's health and welfare.[2]

The health of schoolchildren was also an educational concern, for ill and malnourished children were unable to take full advantage of the free education that more and more states were requiring by law. "From the educational point of view," noted one home economist, "repeated experiments have conclusively proved that it is the well-nourished children who take high rank in education and that it is the army of the under-fed that hold back the efficiency of our public schools. It is costly to educate a child, and the cost is certainly wasted if the system instructs those who are dull because of improper feeding."[3] Despite the confidence with which health experts drew a direct connection between the belly and the brain, there were no scientific studies in the early twentieth century that demonstrated a correlation between nutritional health and academic performance.[4] But teachers and medical inspectors across the country routinely reported that malnourished children were more likely to be absent, tardy, inattentive, apathetic, and generally unable to benefit from educational efforts, and they seemed to succumb more readily to infectious diseases. This experience, even in the absence of definitive studies, contributed to the emergence of a powerful narrative about the relationship between diet, health, behavior, and academic achievement.

In response to concerns about child hunger, malnutrition, and generally poor health, the feeding of schoolchildren became an increasingly central topic in discussions of the role and responsibilities of American public schools. By the first decade of the twentieth century, a reform movement was coalescing around the promotion of public health nutrition and the need for schools to support children's nutritional health. Educators, physicians, nurses, home economists, nutritionists, and philanthropists in cities across the United States began advocating for meal programs, in part to address the logistical challenges of educating children away from home and in part to address the sociomedical problems of hunger and malnourishment. School breakfasts and lunches, milk programs, and similar endeavors thus emerged alongside other expansions and innovations in school health work, including medical inspection, school nurses, playgrounds and outdoor recreation, instruction in health and hygiene, open-air classrooms, and separate classes for children with disabilities or special needs.[5]

As with many public health innovations in this era, American cities trailed their European counterparts in establishing school meal programs. In 1882, Paris became the first major city to provide meals to schoolchildren at public expense. By the first decade of the twentieth century, England, France, Holland, Norway, Sweden, and Switzerland had passed national legislation authorizing school authorities to provide meals in schools using public funds, and local initiatives were common in Belgium, Denmark, Germany, and Italy.[6]

While European measures to feed schoolchildren generally predated American attempts to do the same, there were several important differences between school meal programs as they were conceived and developed on opposite sides of the Atlantic. First, European meal programs generally followed from the assumption that with state-mandated education came state responsibility for the health of schoolchildren. This was a far more contentious position in the United States, where even many proponents of school meals took pains to insist that responsibility for feeding children remained with the home, that children should pay at least a nominal fee to prevent dependency and pauperization, and that schools were not institutions of charity or social work. The school, in that case, served only a facilitating role, with the result that most of the cost of school meals was typically paid directly by students or defrayed by private donations; the use of public monies was usually restricted to the construction and maintenance of facilities and, in some cases, the salaries of personnel.

Second, oversight of American education fell under the purview of the states, not the federal government, which meant that school meal programs were locally established and managed. Because virtually no states explicitly authorized such programs, leaving them in something of a legal gray area, they were often established and managed by private entities such as women's clubs, parent-teacher associations, or other community organizations. Federal support for school meals in the United States ultimately came only as an emergency response to the deprivations of the Great Depression, and there was no permanent, national legislation authorizing the provision of meals with public funds until 1946—and that legislation was an entitlement, not a mandate. Thus the availability, conduct, cost, and quality of school meals in the United States varied substantially from city to city, and even across schools within the same city. In some cases, this meant that those who needed nutritional assistance most were least likely to get it, as in cities with segregated school systems or stark socioeconomic divides.

Yet the circumstances that led to the development of school meal programs in Europe were largely the same as those pressuring the United States: industrialization, urbanization, growing opposition to child labor, increased state involvement in social welfare and public health, and, perhaps most important, passage of compulsory education laws.[7] Massachusetts was the first state to pass a compulsory education law (1852), and all forty-eight states had done so by 1918. By requiring children to attend school, state lawmakers facilitated the expansion of state influence over children, families, and communities. Requiring attendance at school and enforcing it through truancy officers and work permits led to state involvement in matters not only of education but also of health, labor, welfare, and other once-private domains. By the turn of the twentieth century, the school had transformed into a central civic and social institution, a key venue for state interaction with children and their families and public intervention in private affairs. This redefined the boundaries between home and state, and between private rights and public welfare.[8]

Compulsory education placed school-aged children under the supervision of the state, literally and figuratively, facilitating the establishment and rapid growth of routine and widespread health surveillance. Only one U.S. city had regular school medical inspection in 1890, but more than four hundred did by 1910, bringing millions of children into contact with health authorities for the first time.[9] Physicians and nurses working in the schools documented numerous health problems. Although the most common—including poor eyesight, postural disorders, and carious teeth—were relatively minor, many were not so benign, and health problems were identified in a shockingly high number of children; according to one national review, as many as 75 percent of schoolchildren bore at least one physical or mental "defect," many of which were attributed to malnourishment and other remediable conditions.[10] School medical inspection marked the first time that such large numbers of children were examined regularly by nurses and physicians, and the examinations revealed the pervasiveness of both acute and chronic child health problems.

At the same time, exposés by journalists, settlement workers, and social reformers—including Jacob Riis's *How the Other Half Lives* (1890), Robert Hunter's *Poverty* (1904), Upton Sinclair's *The Jungle* (1906), and John Spargo's *Underfed Schoolchildren* (1906)—depicted the devastating toll that steady immigration, rapid industrialization, and brutal labor practices were exacting on people living and working in densely populated cities. Against the backdrop of diminishing infant mortality rates, substantial reductions in major epidemic diseases, improved municipal sanitation, and effective treatments for common childhood diseases like diphtheria, the poor health of American children in the early twentieth century was a shock to health experts and the public alike, the more so because Americans were assumed to be taller and heavier on average—and thus healthier and better fed—than their European counterparts.[11]

The revelations of widespread ill health and poor physical condition among children and young adults in American cities led many to advocate for school-based health services, including school nurses, physical education and outdoor play, dental clinics, special classes for disabled or tubercular children, and school meal programs. "It may be as much the duty of the state to supplement at school the insufficient and wrong feeding in the homes," argued a teacher from Boston, "as it is to supply the instruction which the parents are unable to give."[12]

But the justifications given for the importance of school meal programs were varied, reflecting different ideological and professional perspectives. Arguments from *morality* defined access to sufficient (or sufficiently nourishing) food as a human right, obliging the state to ensure that children were adequately fed. Arguments from *economy* stressed that well-fed children were easier and less expensive to educate, and that they grew up to become better workers, soldiers, and mothers. Arguments from *prophylaxis* suggested that well-nourished children succumbed with less frequency to infectious diseases (thus stemming dissemination) and were less likely to suffer stunted growth, developmental problems, and disability. Feeding children in school would thus lower the incidences of acute and chronic health issues, not only among the malnourished but in the school-aged population as a whole. Of course, these three categories were not mutually exclusive; though separable conceptually, they were often intertwined in actual usage.

The argument for state intervention in schoolchildren's health based on morality, an evocation of health as a basic human right, coincided with larger social changes in the value of children. With declines in both average family size and infant mortality rates, along with a shift toward urban living—where children were more expensive and less able to contribute to the livelihood of the family[13]—children became "emotionally priceless" rather than economically valuable. Over the first decades of the twentieth century, as the sociologist Viviana Zelizer has shown, children's lives became "sacred"; the death of a child was "an intolerable sacrilege, provoking not only parental sorrow but social bereavement as well."[14] In this context, the health of children was as much an ethical issue as a practical one. "It is less a question of parental responsibility than of children's rights," wrote Ernest Hoag and Lewis Terman of school health services in 1914. "Least of all need we prematurely be frightened by the specter of socialism. To protect the bodies of children from defective development is not a question of socialism, but of humanity and of common sense."[15] Hoag, then medical director of the Long Beach City Schools in California, and Terman, a child psychologist and professor of education at Stanford University, framed the issue of school health as an issue of children's rights. The state thus had a moral duty to protect and maintain the health of schoolchildren.

In his work on school reform in the Progressive Era, the historian William Reese has shown that the platform advocating school meals and other children's health initiatives as fundamental rights united socialists, labor groups, social Christians, grassroots activists, and other reformers.[16] For many in this coalition, it was the state's responsibility not only to ensure that schoolchildren were well fed but to provide meals free of charge to those who needed them; it was not enough to give students the opportunity to purchase food from a private, profiting vendor, as was already common in some high schools by the first decade of the twentieth century. High schools, which were not as numerous as elementary schools and thus often farther from children's homes, began lunch programs as a matter more of convenience than of public health or social welfare, and their student bodies included few children from the poorer classes.

Although the moral argument was persuasive in some contexts, its association with socialism (whether explicit or tacit) and confusion with charity or poor relief weakened its influence with school boards and state legislatures—most of which were composed largely of conservative men. Free school meals, like many other aspects of state-funded social welfare, challenged the liberalist ethic of self-determination and personal responsibility, and they raised concerns among the upper classes about the cultivation of dependency and pauperization in the lower classes.

But while the argument for free meals generally found little traction with boards of education, the argument that the state should take more responsibility for children's health and welfare was more successful, particularly when couched in terms of economic success and national strength. S. Josephine Baker, director of the Bureau of Child Hygiene in the New York City Health Department, noted in 1918 that people had "become used to the trite expressions that 'the child is the ward of the state' and that 'the child is the asset of the next generation.'"[17] Many reformers found that emphasizing the economy of feeding schoolchildren, rather than social justice, children's rights, or democratic egalitarianism, tended to have more influence with education leaders, politicians, and others in positions of power. "Boards of education are considering the problem from the economic viewpoint," the Ohio State University Extension Service claimed, "because there seems to be a relation between malnutrition and retardation in school. A poorly nourished child is an economic liability in any school system."[18] Charged with educating children at public expense, education authorities were concerned that malnutrition and other health problems would slow or even prevent students' developmental and academic progress.

"The expensive machinery of education is wasted," argued Mary Swartz Rose, professor of nutrition at Columbia University's Teachers College, "when it operates on a mind listless from hunger or befogged by indigestible food."[19] That expensive machinery was the central concern of school authorities, and its efficient operation their primary goal. Principles of scientific management and corporate efficiency, as espoused by Frederick Taylor and Henry Ford, focused attention on processes and the important role of managers. From the standpoint of educational management, if hunger and malnutrition were preventing the proper education and development of children into healthy, productive adults, school meals could be a viable method for improving the economy of schooling. But by that reasoning, making meals available to all children—especially if offered free of charge—was simply wasteful. Thus the economic argument was to some extent incommensurate with the argument that *all* children have a right to be sufficiently and properly fed.

Arguments based on the economic advantages of school meals also stressed that feeding children would prevent degeneration, both physical and moral. "Every dollar so expended," claimed one physician, "will later be saved in diminished cost of supporting courts, reformatories, alms-houses and jails."[20] The pediatrician Ira Wile concurred: "It is cheaper to feed a child in school than in a hospital or in a prison."[21] Such arguments echoed eugenic and social Darwinian narratives of degeneracy and race suicide, in which social problems such as poverty and crime were explained by hereditary mechanisms,[22] but also challenged them, asserting that physical weakness and immorality were products of environment, not heredity. "On all sides we hear about race suicide," wrote one commentator in 1910,

> and we have it drilled into our ears that the nation whose birth rate decreases is well started on the road that leads to degeneration. To all of this everybody is constantly saying "Amen" with pious fervor. Meanwhile what children there are in the country

may die from malnutrition without anybody becoming particularly excited over the fact. . . . It would really seem to an impartial observer from Mars or some other logically minded planet that we ought either to take care of the children when they are here or else drown them as soon as they are born.[23]

In this *euthenic* framework, the solution to problems of "degeneracy" was better care, not better breeding—and the solution was economically simple: invest now to save later.[24]

Others linked nourishment and physical fitness directly to national interests in advocating for school meals. "The children of to-day," wrote Hoag and Terman, "must be viewed as the raw material of a new State; the schools as the nursery of the Nation."[25] By the first decade of the twentieth century, there was a general preoccupation with the future strength of the country. The expansionist foundations laid during the administration of Benjamin Harrison (1889–1893) had begun a shift in policy from internal annexation and isolationism to foreign intervention and regional hegemony. Fully realized under Theodore Roosevelt, the pursuit of global economic and military advantage through big-stick diplomacy, military incursion, and the aggressive development of favorable foreign markets linked the strength of the nation to the strength of its people. The health of the body was the health of the body politic, and the health of children predicted the health of the future state.[26] "The kind of food a child has to-day," warned Lucy Gillet, a nutritionist at the U.S. Bureau of Education, "determines to a considerable extent the fitness of the future citizen."[27]

But it was not only food that children required. They also needed to learn how to eat for health, growth, and fitness to be of continued value to the state. "The education of the appetite," argued one high school teacher, "may do as much for the future well being of the citizen and for his efficiency in society as the instruction he receives in the mysteries of the 'three R's.'"[28] The New York State Federation of Labor suggested "that there be established in connection with every school a system of furnishing school lunches at a nominal cost for the purpose of demonstrating food values, and thereby assuring us, through educational processes, more healthy men and women in the future."[29] The school meal was not just food but also an edible text, a way of training the mind by nourishing the body. In theory, school meals modeled food consumption according to nutritional principles and influenced the conformation of children's diets with national public health goals beyond school and into adulthood. For most reformers, even many who adopted an economic perspective on the problem, providing meals was but the centerpiece of a fully laden table that would include education in food, nutrition, and cookery; comprehensive health services; research on nutrition health; social work and community outreach; and other services that would address not only children's food intake but the food security and nutritional ecology of entire communities.

Advocates for the importance of school meals also noted a third advantage of school lunches by pointing to the prophylactic benefits of feeding malnourished children. Pediatricians argued that malnutrition led to numerous health problems, including "tuberculosis, adenitis, mental defects, anemia, defects in vision, protracted convalescence from disease, and impaired resistance to the infectious diseases."[30] Feeding children addressed malnutrition directly and numerous other diseases and conditions indirectly. "War on underfeeding and malnutrition needs to be waged even more vigorously than war on typhoid and tuberculosis," argued one nutritionist, "for it is the undernourished, run-down system that is especially susceptible to disease."[31] Preventing and treating malnutrition was a way of limiting numerous other diseases and represented a powerful argument for the importance of ensuring well-nourished schoolchildren. Indeed, anti-tuberculosis associations were some of the most active supporters of school meal programs. The National Tuberculosis Association and local tuberculosis societies, for example, provided financial support for many meal initiatives at regular and open-air schools across the country.

Wile drew an explicit correlation between school meals and medical inspection in their mutual impact on the future health of children.

> The purposes of school lunches and medical inspection are largely identical. Both are designed to act in a preventive and curative way in all phases of physical and mental health. Medical inspection seeks in part to eliminate contagious diseases from

the public schools, while school lunches aim to increase the resistance of children to contagious diseases. Medical inspection seeks out physical and mental defects; school lunches aim to prevent or relieve physical or mental defects. The common ground of school lunches and medical inspection might well be said to be the prevention, determination, and relief of malnutrition.[32]

The school lunch was thus a critical part of school health services more generally, a way to address through one initiative the manifold health problems that beset American children. Without vaccines for every childhood disease, a nutrition vaccination could protect children, and instead of identifying and correcting poor health only after the fact, school meals could reduce the incidence of numerous defects in development and health.

Whether sufficient and complete nourishment was a human right, an economic investment, or a key objective of preventive medicine and public health, there was general agreement that hunger and malnutrition were substantial children's health problems that required some response from the state. "Hunger is a stern condition, not a social theory," the pediatrician and school hygiene specialist Lewis Rapeer argued.

> It cannot be met through the offering of a geography or a grammar. It is clear that where social conditions exist which involve the presence in school of large numbers of unfed or underfed children, it is the function of the school to see to it that some means be provided whereby these children can obtain food in order that they may be in condition to obtain knowledge. This does not necessarily involve provision by the school itself. It does involve the facing of the problem and the securing of some solution for it.[33]

Support for school meals as a solution to this problem was by no means universal; school meals did not so much unite reformers with a wide variety of perspectives and goals as provide a concrete context for the expression and negotiation of various public health, educational, and political agendas, as subsequent chapters explore. But beginning in the last decade of the nineteenth century, a number of community organizations and charitable enterprises began partnering with schools to supply milk, snacks, or meals to urban schoolchildren.

Such initiatives began in the large cities of the North—Boston, Chicago, Cleveland, Cincinnati, Milwaukee, New York, and Philadelphia— and quickly spread throughout the country. The earliest sustained meal programs were organized and operated by community organizations funded by charitable donations: the New England Kitchen, founded by the home economists Ellen Richards and Mary Abel, began preparing lunches in a central kitchen for sale at cost in the high schools of Boston in 1894; that same year, the Starr Center Association began offering penny-portions of soup, cocoa, and crackers to schoolchildren in Philadelphia, and later partnered with the Home and School League to expand the program; and in 1904, the Woman's School Alliance of Milwaukee initiated a service where volunteers, funded by donations from various churches, societies, clubs, and individuals, prepared food in their homes to be given free of charge to needy schoolchildren in three different parts of the city.

Early school meal programs conformed to a commonly employed model of public health development during the Progressive Era, in which private, community-based organizations initiated experimental programs with the hope that, should they prove successful, the programs would be incorporated into publicly funded and managed municipal health services. As the historian Judith Walzer Leavitt has shown in her study of public health in Milwaukee, for example, women's clubs, church groups, settlement houses, and voluntary civic organizations raised money for, and often provided directly, health services for those who could not afford private medical care and could not wait years for the benefits of sanitation and disease control. Yet ultimately, they intended these programs to become a part of the city's public health machinery.[34]

By 1913, just two decades after the first sustained school meal programs were established in the United States, at least forty-six cities had instituted some form of school foodservice, which was quickly becoming a recognizable and widely praised feature of urban public schools. While concern about hunger and malnutrition focused attention on the nutritional health of schoolchildren, there were two additional issues for which school meal programs provided a concrete solution. First, school meal programs addressed the difficulty mothers faced in preparing portable lunches for their children to take to school. Second, school meal programs addressed the risks to children's health—nutritional, bacterial, and chemical—of consuming the ready-to-eat foods becoming widely available from street vendors, restaurants, and other food purveyors in the vicinity of schools.

For many mothers, school meals were not an unwelcome intrusion of the state into private, household affairs but a relief from the laborious and often bewildering task of preparing portable lunches for their children. "It is much more difficult," wrote one mother in the *National Congress of Mothers Magazine,* "to make a luncheon attractive and appetizing when it must be put up, and not eaten for several hours, than it is to serve it on one's table fresh from range or pantry."[35] With larger numbers of children attending school—and larger numbers of mothers joining the urban workforce—providing for children in the middle of the day became a source of stress for many mothers. In Spirit Lake, Iowa, for instance, some said "that they would depend quite largely on the lunch served at school both in the interests of their children's health and as a solution for the lunch box problem, which is not an easy one."[36] Although conservative commentators continued to stress that the care of children in all its aspects was the responsibility of the home, mothers were generally quite happy to see schools assist them with this charge, particularly when it came to providing food during the school day.

Advice on how to pack lunches for schoolchildren was ubiquitous in the popular literature of the early twentieth century. Newspaper and magazine articles contained discussion of every aspect of the portable lunch, including recipes, amounts and kinds of food to include, nutritional contributions of different foods, attractive presentation, packing techniques and materials, and the advantages of different kinds of carrying receptacles. Metal lunch boxes or pails, for example, were superior to baskets because they were durable and easy to clean and disinfect. Nut spreads made a good sandwich filling when meat was not available. The contents of the lunch should be wrapped individually, because this both kept the flavors and aromas from mixing unpleasantly and made the child more likely to eat everything because each part of the lunch was like a small present.[37]

Based on the advice literature, packing a "proper" lunch required knowledge of nutrition and food preparation, time and planning, and appropriate packaging; in the preparation of lunches, mothers were to be part nutritionist, part psychologist, part chef, and part entertainer. Preparing high-quality, nutritious lunches that children would enjoy was also a significant challenge. "Of all the work a mother has to do for her children," wrote one mother in *Harper's Bazaar*, "none is more monotonous, more troublesome, than putting up of lunches day after day, with a due regard for variety and wholesomeness and for the fickle and often unreasonable taste of the child."[38] Making lunches was thus a source of angst for many mothers; it was not only an indication of their fitness as parents but also a key factor in the nutritional health and educational performance of their children, which were routinely evaluated by public health workers and teachers.

School meal programs offered mothers a reprise from the burden of packing lunches. In 1905, after three years of operation, the cafeteria at the Los Angeles Normal School prompted glowing praise from one commentator, who highlighted both its health benefits and the assistance it provided to mothers: "Would it be too much to hope for such a dining-room . . . in every public school building in the city? It might pay in the increased health and strength of the future men and women. And oh! how much worry it would save the mothers in the homes."[39] That worry came not just from the responsibility of ensuring a child's well-being and capacity to learn but also from the constantly changing and often confusing nutritional advice literature. "It is impossible for the busy and often overworked mother to keep abreast of the revolutionary changes that are constantly taking place in this great problem of efficient home-making," observed a journalist in Fresno, California. "This brings the work to the school."[40] Others observed that the labor involved in preparing portable meals was less concerning than the labor it took to digest them. "Pity the woman who must put up a daily lunch for the school boy or girl," noted one advice columnist in the *New York Times*. "That pity is deserved, but far more of it should go to the average victim of those baskets."[41]

For most reformers, school meal programs had the potential to do far more than simply feed children. Ideally, school meals would serve an educational function, too, wherein children would apply the lessons of the lunchroom to their eating habits more broadly and bring their new knowledge of foods and nutrition home to their mothers. "The painstaking work of the school lunch supervisors to secure wholesome and adequate noon meals for the school children at a minimum cost not only brings immediate benefit to the children," argued the nutritionist Mary Rose, "but exerts a widespread influence upon homes and parents, as the children carry to them reports of these concrete lessons in the science of proper selection, preparation, and hygiene of food."[42] Although in most cases this transference was probably minimal, school meals were an effective bridge between home and school, and a demonstration of the role that the public school could play in the health and welfare of both children and their communities. "Far from weakening the sense of responsibility of the home," Cincinnati's superintendent of schools noted in 1912, the city's school meal service had "aroused the interest of the homes in better hygienic conditions and has fostered more intelligent selection and preparation of nourishing foods."[43]

School meals provided a conduit between children and their families, helping to establish the school as a community-based social institution and not merely a place to educate the young. In particular, feeding children in the schools stimulated greater parental involvement in issues of food and nutrition, but also in the school as a whole. After a school feeding experiment conducted by the University of Chicago School of Education in 1920, the researchers noted that "most of the mothers visited the lunch once or twice during the term, and great was their amazement at the amounts of food their children ate, as well as at seeing them eat willingly things they had never touched at home."[44] Similarly, the Northwestern Women's Club initiated a lunch service at the Clinton School in Detroit, and after thirteen weeks, they found the mothers of children there over three times as likely to attend meetings at the school when compared with a school having no lunch program.[45] In Philadelphia, mothers went to the lunchrooms requesting recipes for the dishes served and desiring to purchase the leftovers. Mothers in New York City sometimes bought *their* lunches at the schools, too, even eating with the children on occasion.[46] School meals, proponents argued, stimulated parental involvement both in the school as an institution and in the nutrition problems of children.

Support for school meal programs expanded considerably after the United States entered World War I, in large part because the medical examinations of potential soldiers revealed the widespread and serious consequences of childhood malnourishment. Of the over 3 million young men who applied for military service in 1917–1918, more than 30 percent were rejected on medical grounds, mostly for defects of the heart, eyes, and bones; the fifth leading cause of rejection was underweight, and 8 percent of those rejected for medical reasons suffered from some physical, developmental defect.[47] Surgeon General Rupert Blue and other health authorities drew a clear connection between many of these defects and chronic malnutrition during childhood.[48] Although statisticians and epidemiologists cautioned against exaggerating the importance of the findings—the purpose of the exams was to evaluate men for soldiering, not for basic health—the results revealed extensive disease and disability among men in the prime of life. Nor were such poor results likely limited to men: "No one doubts that if such tests had been made of our young women," remarked Alice Wood, director of a child health organization in Chicago, "even a greater percentage of physical defects and insufficiency would have been disclosed."[49] Awareness of malnutrition as a national health problem spread quickly: one survey of periodic literature found that the number of articles on malnutrition appearing in twenty popular magazines and professional journals rose from an average of just seven per year between 1912 and 1917 to nearly sixty in 1922 alone.[50]

By the 1920s, at least in the popular imagination, the lunch box was becoming a symbol of obsolescence in the rapidly modernizing urban public schools. "The old-fashioned lunch box for school children seems likely to be extinct," claimed one Seattle newspaper. "Instead, [children] line up at noon and file past a cafeteria counter, each carrying a tray, and select with care the articles of food that appeal to them."[51] This view was echoed in Chicago: "Taking its place in the museum of the out-of-date, along with the old oaken bucket, the horsehair sofa, and the patent leather buggy, is the old tin dinner pail that accompanied a child to school. In its place in the schoolhouse is the cafeteria tray loaded with a balanced meal of warm food and milk."[52] Even in smaller cities like Sandusky, Ohio, "the little tin lunch pail and its successor, the fiber lunch box, are passing."[53]

When reformers predicted the extinction of the lunch box and the success of the school lunch, they were envisioning a state in which children's nutritional health was ensured not solely by mothers but also by scientific experts. According to the superintendent of household arts and science at the Mechanics Institute of Rochester, New York, "The lunch box, with its reminiscent odors of pie and pickles and its germ-harboring possibilities, belongs to a domestic science-less past."[54] More than merely teaching mothers how to choose and prepare food, nutritionists and educators sought to undertake those roles themselves, attempting to correct the nutritional problems of the nation by changing the diets of children on a large scale.

Yet mothers were not the only source of lunches for schoolchildren. Instead of bringing food or returning home to eat, many children patronized restaurants, corner stores, bakeries, and street vendors for lunch (see figure 1). The results of this were, according to one Chicago student, "a pain in the stomach, an ache in the head, a zero in the teacher's class-book, and a great daub of blueberry pie on the shirt waist."[55] Educators, nutritionists, and physicians lamented the choices that students made when left to select meals for themselves. Children ate according to taste and not according to the principles of health and nutrition, and they didn't get the maximum nutritive value for their money.

Across the nation, schoolchildren often skipped breakfast, consumption of coffee and tea was common, and pickles, pie, and sweets comprised a great many lunches. In Los Angeles, for example, "ice cream and tamales constitute the 'substantials' on the bill of fare, as of yore, but they do not fill the bill at the noon hour."[56] In Decatur, Illinois, one street vendor claimed that he sold "a barrel of dill pickles a week to the school children," which physicians warned "was not only mildly unhygienic but absolutely ruinous to the health of children."[57] When surveyed about what he had eaten for lunch, one New Haven student wrote: "Bought a dozen crullers. Ate all of them. Bad for the

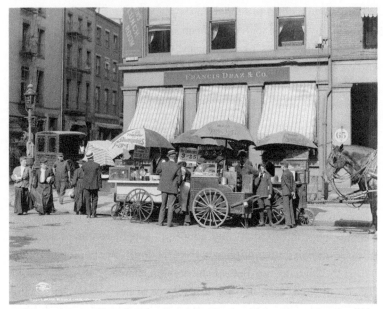

Figure 1. Lunch carts on Broad Street, New York City, c. 1906. (Note also the lunchroom on the second floor of the building in the background.) Industrialization, urbanization, and compulsory education generated a substantial market for ready-to-eat foods.

Source: Library of Congress, LC-D4–19577.

health."[58] Nearly a third of the schoolchildren surveyed in twelve Wisconsin counties drank coffee on a daily basis.[59] The lunches of pupils at PS 1 in Manhattan were "without exception bought from a push-cart or a basket on the curb in front of the schoolhouse. It need not be said that such a luncheon usually consisted of doughnuts, crullers, pretzels and bad, highly-colored, highly-flavored candy."[60] And in San Antonio, vendors came to schools "with wheelbarrows, buggies, baskets, glass-covered stands, wagons, galvanized tin boxes and with every conceivable kind of receptacle," from which were sold "hamburgers, Mexican candies, pies, cakes, sandwiches, fruits, 'hot dogs,' ice cream cones and all the customary 'eat-in-hand' morsels."[61]

Selling food to schoolchildren was big business. In 1913, 170,000 elementary schoolchildren in Philadelphia spent approximately $200,000 on food during school hours, and most of it went to the proprietors of pushcarts and small stores.[62] The semipermanent outdoor stalls of the country's ten largest cities were estimated to be worth $10 million in 1903, and that doesn't include pushcarts, wagons, baskets, and other mobile vending devices. Many street merchants sold foods and drinks to meet the lunch demands not only of schoolchildren but also of the large and growing industrial workforce. Fruit stands were particularly lucrative: a stand that cost $20 to build, operated on space rented for $75 per month, could generate up to $10 a day in profit.[63] "It is difficult to determine what is not sold in the eatable and drinkable line at these primitive lunch counters," observed a police officer in Cleveland. "Oysters, clams, fishballs, meat cakes, sausages, cold meats, sandwiches, fried fish, fried potatoes, pretzels, pies, rolls, buttermilk, sweet milk, lemonade, coffee, tea, root beer and orangeade are only a few of the refreshments to be purchased, and everything is as cheap as dirt."[64] The growing market on city streets for candy, ice cream, soft drinks, and other sweets reflected larger changes in dietary patterns: candy consumption rose from 2.2 pounds per capita in 1880 to 13.1 in 1919 (a sixfold increase), and ice cream consumption increased from 1.5 pounds per capita in 1909 to 7.5 in 1920 (a fivefold increase).[65]

Concerns about street foods were not solely nutritional. When local health departments and the USDA began chemical and bacteriological analyses of foods in the late nineteenth century, they found high rates of adulteration. Ground meats, as found in the popular sausages and frankfurters, often contained chemical preservatives used to pass off tainted meat as edible; breads and cakes contained sawdust, chalk, or clay to increase their weight; milk was found to be diluted with water or sourced from diseased cows; and numerous other foodstuffs contained high levels of dangerous chemicals and bacteria. In chocolate, for example, chemists found powdered soap, beans, and peas, to which the makers added red oxide of mercury, a lethal toxin in large amounts, in order to restore the chocolate's dark color.[66]

The premises on which these foods were prepared and served—and the people who prepared and served them—were seen as an additional health hazard in the urban market for ready-to-eat meals. The food sold by street vendors was "unsanitary and unwholesome," according to one nutritionist, due as much to the conditions of preparation and sale as to the race of the vendors. "It is carried to the school in open wagons or push carts, exposed to dust and flies and the dirty hands of the dealers, until, from the standpoint of sanitation alone, it is a real menace to health. It is, with few exceptions, prepared and sold by ignorant people—Mexicans, negroes and the like."[67] In the city of Chicago, thousands of saloons offered free lunches to entice customers. Prior to 1915, the Health Department's Bureau of Food Inspection lacked the authority to regulate foodservice in saloons, where the utensils and dishes were reused by numerous customers without washing and the kitchens often fell far short of the hygienic standards to which restaurant kitchens were held.[68] To the urban worker or schoolchild, street foods offered seemingly endless variety, exceptionally low prices, and a hot meal even away from home. But to the nutritionist or health officer, street foods—often adulterated, contaminated, and lacking in nutrients—were a substantial risk to health.

Given this situation, one may wonder why students weren't simply prohibited from leaving school grounds, as is common practice today, to prevent them from purchasing lunch from street vendors and local stores or restaurants. While a few schools took this approach, it was not a common one, and those that did were all high schools. Attendance at school was not required by law after the eighth grade, which gave high schools more latitude to impose restrictions on students. In addition, the practice of allowing elementary schoolchildren to return home for lunch was widely accepted—how could the state deny the right of parents to feed their children at home, especially in the context of widespread concern over malnourishment? Schools in this period had not yet attained the expansive social authority over children's activities that they would later in the century.

Yet as nutritionists and home economists, physicians and nurses, clubwomen and philanthropists, and in some cases school boards and state legislators sought to establish school meal programs for the first time, they faced numerous obstacles—social, political, legal, economic, and logistical. The next three chapters explore in depth the efforts to establish school meal programs in three different contexts. Each of the three case studies highlights a different aspect of the challenges that beset establishment of permanent, publicly funded meal programs. Chapter 2 uses the city of Chicago's efforts to create a school meal service to explore the legal ambiguity that attended the use of public monies to feed of schoolchildren. Chapter 3 examines the case of New York City, where sociopolitical resistance to expanding the roles and responsibilities of the public schools clashed with a vocal lobby for the importance of school lunches as a civic service and public health initiative. Chapter 4 then moves from the city to the country, where efforts to feed children were hampered far more by logistical and geographic constraints than by ideological ones. Collectively, these chapters reveal how social, political, and ecological factors shaped the form and function of school meal programs.

Chapter 2

(Il)Legal Lunches

School Meals in Chicago

In 1908, the Chicago Board of Education estimated that of the 300,000 children attending public schools, nearly 5,000 were "habitually hungry," upward of 15,000 were not receiving "three square meals daily," and over 30,000 needed more food.[1] At the Oliver Goldsmith School in the Jewish Ghetto,[2] for example, 5 percent of the children arrived at school without having eaten breakfast. According to the school's principal:

> Unquestionably a majority of the children attending this school are improperly fed, especially in the lower grades. . . . When I began work here I discovered that many of the pupils remained all day without food. A great majority of the parents in this district, as well as the older children, are at work from dawn to dusk, and have no time to care for the little ones. Such children have no place to go when dismissed at noon, and are usually back at the school building within ten minutes.[3]

Moreover, medical inspectors found that nearly half of Chicago's school children suffered from one or more physical defects, many of which resulted from chronic malnourishment.[4]

Concerned about the health and education of malnourished children, the Board of Education proposed to use public funds to provide free midmorning meals in the public schools. When the board sought community input on the plan, parents—especially poor, widowed, and single mothers—responded enthusiastically and "welcomed it as a helping hand." Middle-class charity workers, however, soundly rejected it. "Under normal conditions 90 per cent of our people are able to care for their children and do so," Othelia Myhrman of the Swedish National Association reported. "We do not believe that a school breakfast in the largest number of cases would be of any great benefit." T. D. Hurley, president of the Visitation Aid Society, claimed that providing free breakfasts would "do lasting harm to parents and children by making them dependent." The Jewish Aid Society echoed this view: "If any of the Jewish children go to school hungry, it is unnecessary, and the parents should be dealt with and compelled to do their duty, instead of being made even more dependent than they already are."[5]

For the city's charity workers, malnourished children were a private, not a public, responsibility; for public officials, this amounted to a denial of the problem. Assistant County Agent Victor Young observed that "private charity seems to have made up a case against the proposition that a large number of children are going to school hungry. My experience leads me to believe that this is a fact and an impressive one." Superintendent of Schools W. L. Bodine agreed, reporting to the Board of Education that tens of thousands of Chicago children were unable to benefit from free public education because they were so poorly nourished. Commissioner of Health W. A. Evans, dismayed at the findings of school medical inspectors, established a corps of forty school nurses to address the poor health of the city's youth.[6] Despite the testimony of school and health officials, middle-class charity workers feared that excessive public intervention would lead to dependency and pauperization among the poor, and they opposed the proposal for a publicly funded meal program. The problem was not that the Board of Education wanted to provide food for children but that it proposed doing so at public expense. This proposition, which was characterized as socialist, threatened to make the school an institution of social welfare rather than of education; for Chicago's aid societies, those two functions were incommensurate.

The dominant model of charity in the early twentieth century remained a strictly hierarchical one, in which class and wealth determined responsibility. "The duty of the man of wealth," argued the steel magnate Andrew Carnegie in his 1889 essay "The Gospel of Wealth," is "to consider all surplus revenues which come to him simply as trust funds," which he should administer so as "to produce the most beneficial results for the community."[7] Charity organization societies, of which there were upward of one hundred by the turn of the century, acted as brokers between the rich and the poor, ensuring that such relief was well spent and aided only the "deserving poor," those who were not indolent, intemperate, or immoral. Most importantly, this system was entirely private; middle-class charity workers solicited money from the wealthy to be rationally administered on behalf of the poor, all without the expenditure of public funds or involvement of public agencies.[8]

Chicago was unusual in that the Board of Education took an active role in the development of a school meal program. In most cities, such initiatives followed the charity model: they emerged from the work of private organizations and only later became a function of public agencies. The New England Kitchen and the Women's Educational and Industrial Union in Boston, the Starr Center Association and the Home and School League in Philadelphia, the Woman's School Alliance in Milwaukee, and the School Lunch Committee in New York City all developed school meal services independently, using private funds, with the ultimate goal of transferring the work to the city. This was a traditional process, not only for school meal programs but for many other public health initiatives, such as visiting nurses or community health centers. Private organizations innovated on a small scale, then transferred successful programs to public agencies, which implemented them on a large scale. This system, the historian Judith Walzer Leavitt has argued in her work on public health in Milwaukee, "freed the private agencies to expand their programs in new directions and allowed the health department to broaden and centralize services," creating "channels through which public and private activity could be unified in a single quest for improving citizen health."[9]

Schools present something of a special case in that they blurred the differences between public and private. With community-based health initiatives, private organizations acted as a bridge between the communities with whom they worked and the impersonal bureaucracies of increasingly crowded and fragmented cities. With school-based health initiatives, in contrast, it was often public servants—teachers, principals, school nurses, medical inspectors, and superintendents—who bridged the gap between communities and the state. When community organizations worked through the schools, the services provided, even those entirely funded with private monies, received implicit state endorsement. And schools themselves were community institutions as much as state ones. By the twentieth century, public schools had become the grounds, both literally and figuratively, on which negotiations of public and private responsibility for the health and welfare of children took place.

In Chicago, the debate over publicly funded school meal programs reflected widespread disagreement about the distribution of responsibility for children's health and the proper role of the public schools. In proposing to feed children at public expense, the Board of Education raised two interrelated questions: To what extent should the state assume responsibility for the nutritional health of children, and should the provision of food be a justifiable activity (or expense) for an educational institution? As the board pursued the possibility of providing free meals in the city's schools, these questions shaped the nature of the programs that evolved over the following three decades.

When the Board of Education proposed in 1908 to serve free meals in the public schools, school authorities had not anticipated the resistance of the city's charity workers. Even supporters of the plan worried about the expenditure of public monies for the relief of hunger and malnourishment. Earl Barnes, a prominent professor of education who spoke at a meeting between the Board of Health, the Board of Education, and interested community members, observed that "if you have $3 to spend on a child's education, you had better spend $1.50 for food. You will get better results. The problem is how to feed the child without state socialism and degradation."[10]

This concern that free school meals was a step toward socialism was not strictly ideological; it was also legal. Like public health, education fell under the purview of the states, and the powers of school boards were established by state legislatures and interpreted by the courts. In 1908, no state legislature had specifically authorized boards of education to serve meals, let alone serve them at public expense. Although most school boards had considerable discretion to manage schooling and to disburse school funds as they saw fit, meal programs such as the one proposed by Chicago's Board of Education had no clear legal status. The development of such programs thus occurred not only in lunchrooms but also in courtrooms.

The legal status of providing food for children at public expense was murky at best. On one hand, the Illinois legislature had imbued the board with fairly broad and unrestrictive powers. As one Illinois state judge noted in a 1904 case:

> The [Chicago] board of education is vested with authority in law to take all necessary steps to provide a complete and efficient system of free public schools. This broad law justifies the board in taking whatever action is necessary in relation to broadening the scope of school work. The constitutional provision for a school system confers great powers on boards of education, and I believe intentionally was made as broad as it could be.[11]

States typically granted considerable discretion to school boards in deciding how best to carry out, and even "broaden," their educational mission. On the other hand, the board received a cautionary opinion from its own legal counsel: "It is frequently a very difficult matter to state clearly just what is an educational purpose for which the expenditure of public money will be justified," Frank Hamlin told the board in 1908. "I do not think there can be any question, however, about the fact that it would not be lawful for the Board of Education to undertake the feeding of children directly, and to expend money for that purpose."[12]

Opinions expressing concern about the legality of publicly funded meal programs were not uncommon in the early twentieth century, but Hamlin's was especially restrictive. For example, when the St. Louis Board of Education requested an opinion on the legality of supporting a lunch service in the Central High School in 1903, its attorney F. N. Judson argued that given the distance many students traveled between home and school, it was "a reasonable and proper action on the part of the Board" to establish a department to administer a lunch program. As long as the board did not provide meals free of charge, he continued, the plan would be "free from any objection, and in my opinion does not violate the character or rules of the Board. The fact that experience may develop a deficit which would require an appropriation from the Board to make good in the operation of this department, constitutes no objection, as such a deficit would be clearly incidental."[13] In other words, the Board of Education could not provide free meals, but it could subsidize a lunch program in which the receipts didn't entirely cover expenditures.

The issue, as most legal authorities framed it, was not about whether school boards could *operate* school lunch programs but whether (or to what extent) they could *subsidize* them. Lacking specific authorization from state legislatures, this created a de facto separation of public and private responsibilities. School authorities could provide equipment, water, power, and other infrastructural support, as maintenance and operation of facilities were explicitly assigned to school boards in most cases. In contrast, the purchase of food remained a solidly private responsibility. Underwriting the cost of feeding children directly was widely regarded as beyond the powers of school boards. Labor costs tended to fall somewhere in the middle: some school systems paid dietitians, cooks, or servers out of public funds; others did not. This created incentives for cooperation between public and private entities: private organizations could not retrofit schools for foodservice, and most boards of education could not subsidize meals with public funds.

Despite the implicit legal restrictions, Chicago developed the most extensive school meal program in the country. By 1933, sixty-eight public elementary schools (roughly a quarter of the total) and all fifty-two high schools were serving low-cost meals every school day. The Board of Education managed this by working with Chicago's women's clubs to provide what the schools could not, thus circumventing the perceived legal restrictions.

The Women's Clubs of Chicago, a loosely knit organization that coordinated efforts among the hundreds of women's clubs throughout the city, formed the Chicago School Extension Committee (CSEC) in 1909.[14] The mission of the CSEC, whose members included delegates from a number of independent clubs, was to facilitate collaboration between the Board of Education, individual schools, and interested community leaders to improve conditions in Chicago's public schools, especially the elementary schools. The CSEC worked for the construction of playgrounds, advocated for vacation schools, and sold one-penny bottles of milk to schoolchildren. The CSEC was both an executive committee on schools for members of over seventy women's clubs in Chicago, organizing and concentrating their individual efforts, and also a visible, accessible association to which school authorities could appeal for assistance whenever necessary.

In 1911, Superintendent of Schools Ella Flagg Young requested that the CSEC consider "the feasibility of conducting 'penny lunches' in the public schools, in co-operation with the Board of Education."[15] Though she stood barely five feet tall, Young's imposing intellect and fearless stewardship of Chicago's public schools had earned her the admiration of such luminaries as John Dewey, who regarded her as one "whose experience and advice were invaluable to him," as well as the respect of teachers who "flocked to her lectures."[16] In her more than fifty years as an educator in Chicago, Young installed playground apparatus and promoted the school as a social and community center; she expanded traditional classroom subjects, adding science, hygiene, social studies, and industrial arts to the curriculum; she organized and founded the first school libraries; and she ushered in the city's first open-air school and the first special education school for disabled children.[17] The Chicago Board of Education appointed her superintendent of schools in 1909, and she became the first woman in the country to head a major school system.

As superintendent, Young held the highest administrative position in the Department of Education. She reported directly to the Board of Education and was responsible for the implementation of policy, the hiring and firing of administrators, the oversight of school construction and maintenance, public relations, and the general management of daily operations. She used her office to advocate for the welfare of children, arguing that the schools should be institutions of social betterment, both for the pupils attending them and for the communities supporting them.

In response to Young's proposition, the CSEC suggested that the Board of Education pay the salaries of the lunchroom attendants, supply the permanent equipment, and provide clean rooms for cooking, serving, and dining. The CSEC, in turn, would select the menu, buy and prepare the food, do the accounting, and pay the salary of a "trained supervisor." The CSEC also proposed that each portion of food on the school menu be sold for one cent, making the program accessible even to very poor children. The board unanimously approved the proposal.[18]

This type of relationship—between a municipal institution and a community organization—had several advantages for the Board of Education. Most importantly, it sidestepped any concerns about the legality of feeding children with public money; although the partnership involved some financial contributions from the board, the outlays were minimal and limited. Equipping a school to serve simple meals was relatively inexpensive; out of the roughly $500,000 allotted each year for the construction and maintenance of school buildings and grounds, a one-time expenditure of about $1,000 was usually sufficient to outfit a school kitchen and lunchroom. Instead of simply licensing women's clubs to operate as concessionaires, the collaboration proposed by Young and the CSEC gave the board oversight of day-to-day operations, the ability to negotiate meal prices, and the opportunity to shape the development of school meal programs.

In 1911, three Chicago elementary schools—Adams, Foster, and Jackson—began serving penny lunches daily. These three schools educated children in some of the roughest and most impoverished neighborhoods in the city.

Adams Elementary (Townsend Street, between West Chicago Avenue and Locust Street) served the south side of Little Hell, a badly crowded neighborhood composed largely of Irish, German, and Scandinavian laborers, most of whom toiled in the gas works, and of Sicilian immigrants who grew steadily in number after the turn of the century. Little Hell earned its moniker because the riverside neighborhood had so many alleys and back streets that it became a haven for crime and gang activity. The intersection of Milton and Oak Streets (just two blocks from the Adams School) was dubbed "Death Corner" because of the large number of murders that occurred in the vicinity; between 1910 and 1915, more than 150 people were slain in an area less than ten blocks square.[19]

Foster Elementary (Union Avenue and O'Brien Street) lay at the heart of the Jewish Ghetto. Settled largely by Russian, Polish, and Romanian Jews, the Ghetto was one of the poorest and most crowded neighborhoods in the city. One observer remarked that the residents spent their days in "factories and houses in which many people would not allow a horse to live." The Ghetto also had badly overcrowded schools; each of the eleven schools in the neighborhood had upward of 1,000 enrolled pupils, but most of the buildings had been built to accommodate far fewer.[20]

Andrew Jackson Elementary (Sholto Street between Good and Better Streets) served Little Italy, a district on the Near West Side whose twenty-room school was unable to admit even half of the more than 2,000 enrolled students. One reporter observed that "Little Italy is the city of the children, . . . a city that is crowded—yes, overcrowded— with youngsters, children little, children big, children romping, children working, children laughing, children crying, but all of them extremely dirty."[21] The overcrowding of the schools in this area was due in large part to the pace of Italian immigration. Chicago had only 1,400 Italian immigrants in 1880 but nearly 50,000 by 1910. The Jackson School served an area settled primarily by immigrants from Sicily, Naples, and Messini, and to a lesser extent Genoa, many of whom provided unskilled labor in rail yards and construction sites. This was some of the most demanding and ill-paying work in the city; railroad labor paid $1.50 per twelve-hour shift at a time when it cost around $3.00 per week to rent a tenement apartment.[22]

In the first week of operation, the CSEC served meals to 652 children at the three schools; many more children desired meals, but accommodations were modest at first. At the Jackson School in Little Italy, demand was so great that the lunchroom attendants had to turn away as many as 500 pupils a day.[23] To make the lunches appealing, the CSEC attempted to vary the menus "as much as possible, not only to prevent the children from tiring of the food, but also to cater to the children's tastes in different localities and to acquaint them with different kinds of food that they in turn may urge the use and preparation of similar cheap and nourishing foods at home."[24]

Reflecting national trends, Chicago schools attempted to respect children's religious and cultural preferences when planning meals. Providing foods that did not interfere with religious practices ensured that all children could partake. Out of respect for Catholic tradition, "meat soups are never served on Friday, but cocoa is served instead, in all centers. Also in the Ghetto district the cooking is always done by a 'Kosher' cook." The menus also reflected the ethnicities of the children. "Tomato and macaroni soup will always call a larger number to lunch in the Italian district and the odor of sausage cooking in the Ghetto district has the same effect."[25] The CSEC's attentiveness to the tastes of children in different neighborhoods helped to ensure the popularity, and therefore the success, of the pilot penny lunch programs.

According to the agreement between the Board of Education and the CSEC, each penny portion of food had to provide a minimum of 300 calories, and the cost of a portion was not to exceed one cent on average.[26] By the nutritional standards of the time, children aged six to twelve needed to consume 1,650 to 1,800 calories daily, so the penny portions were not a full meal; children could either purchase one portion as a supplement to food brought from home or buy two portions for a complete meal.[27] Although the menus were typically simple, including sandwiches, soups, bread, milk, and cocoa, children could purchase a complete, nutritious meal for two or three cents.

After the first year, the records of the principals in the three schools showed "less sickness and better daily attendance." According to District Superintendent Minnie Cowan, "Reports from the schools in which the penny lunches have been served for a year or more are most satisfactory, and no argument is needed to convince the community of the advantage [of school lunches]."[28] Feeding children one-cent portions of nourishing food improved the health of children and the effectiveness of the educational process, so the Board of Education and the CSEC expanded the penny lunch program to include more schools.

The CSEC incorporated in 1913, becoming a permanent committee of the Women's Clubs of Chicago, with centralized leadership and delegate members from participating women's clubs. The committee then established penny lunches in eleven more elementary schools, and during the 1913–1914 school year, the CSEC served more than 130,000 lunches in fourteen schools.[29] For its part, the Board of Education continued to equip schools with the necessary apparatus, pay the salaries of lunchroom attendants, and perform routine health inspections. According to section 286 of the Rules of the Board of Education, "Once every two months there shall be an inspection of these lunch rooms by the head of the Department of Domestic Science or some other suitable person ... who shall file with the Superintendent for his approval a report concerning the service given, the quality of the food offered, the price at which it is sold, and the sanitary conditions of these lunch rooms."[30] The partnership between the board and the CSEC provided tens of thousands of children with food that was both nourishing and appetizing by combining the resources and flexibility of a private organization with the stability and accountability of a public institution.

In November of 1914, CSEC members Florence Vosbrink and Hilga Sethness visited the schools with penny lunches to assess how well the program was working; all the principals agreed that "attendance is larger, there is a decrease in epidemics, and children's diseases are less." They also called on eleven schools "in exceedingly poor districts" that did not yet have penny lunches and determined that "lack of food was the cause of many of the absences."[31] In 1915, the Board of Education approved twelve new schools for penny lunch programs, and by 1917, twenty-six elementary schools had them.[32]

As the penny lunch program in the elementary schools continued to expand, Superintendent of Schools John Shoop, who had succeeded Young, proposed in 1917 that the price of the penny lunches be raised to two or three cents per portion. Beginning in the 1910s, the price of food in the United States had increased at a much faster rate than wages and revenue, and he worried that the programs would not remain self-sustaining if children paid only one penny per portion. The board, however, remained committed to keeping prices low. "The board of education wastes enough money without economizing on the children of the poor," President of the Board Jacob Loeb declared. "I

believe proper food is more essential to the school children than reading and arithmetic."[33] The price of a portion of food remained one
cent for a short time, but after American entry into World War I, it
increased to two cents to prevent insolvency due to higher food prices.
The increase did not affect participation, and demand remained high
during and after the war.

With the continued success of the penny lunches, the Board of
Education again investigated the legal status of subsidizing meals in
the schools with public funds, in the hopes of assuming full responsibility for the penny lunch programs. Its attorney Charles Francis gave
much the same opinion as Hamlin had nine years earlier. Although
as yet there was no legal precedent specific to school meal programs,
Francis cited Illinois Supreme Court cases *Wells v. People* (71 Ill. 532),
Peers v. Board of Education (72 Ill. 511), and *School Directors v. Fogel-
man* (76 Ill. 191), as well as the Illinois Appellate Court case *Harris v.
Kill* (108 Ill. App. 305), which limited the executive powers of boards
of education to those expressly granted by the state legislature.[34] However, the state had delineated those powers in laws written decades
earlier, before meals had become a prominent feature of modern
schooling. The 1889 Act to Establish and Maintain a System of Free
Schools, along with amendments passed in 1893, contained the principal laws governing the extent and limitations of the board's powers.
While these included, for example, the duty "to repair and improve
school houses and furnish them with the necessary fixtures, furniture,
apparatus, libraries, and fuel," enabling the board to equip school
kitchens, the laws said nothing about providing food for students.[35]

Francis knew of only one case in which the Illinois Supreme
Court had given any opinion related to the legal right of a school board
to utilize public funds for the provision of food. In the 1873 case *Sher-
lock v. Village of Winnetka* (66 Ill. 530), the court decided that a board
of education could not appropriate funds for the construction of a
boardinghouse or contribute to the cost of boarding—including feeding—students.[36] Other cases were even more restrictive. The Illinois
Appellate Court ruled in *Mills v. School Directors* (154 Ill. App. 119)
"that to secure the right and opportunity of equal education does not
require that the children should be hauled to school, any more than it

would require that the directors should clothe them or furnish meals."
The Illinois Supreme Court also declared unequivocally in *Scown v.
Czarnecki* (264 Ill. 313) that "the public school system of the State was
not established and has not been maintained as a charity or from philanthropic motives."[37] The state attorney general, Edward Brundage,
concurred with the prevailing legal opinion on apportioning public
monies for school meals: "I gravely doubt whether the Board of Education has such right and power."[38]

As late as 1937, twenty years after Francis delivered his report in
Chicago, only sixteen states had passed laws specifically empowering
boards of education to finance and operate lunchrooms in public schools,
and most were quite restrictive (see figure 2).[39] Fear of socializing what

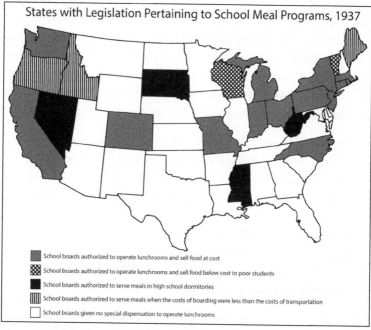

States with Legislation Pertaining to School Meal Programs, 1937

School boards authorized to operate lunchrooms and sell food at cost

School boards authorized to operate lunchrooms and sell food below cost to poor students

School boards authorized to serve meals in high school dormitories

School boards authorized to serve meals when the costs of boarding were less than the costs of transportation

School boards given no special dispensation to operate lunchrooms

Figure 2. American states that sanctioned boards of education to serve food
in public schools as of 1937.

Sources: Everett C. Preston, *Principles and Statutory Provisions Relating to Recreational,
Medical, and Social Welfare Services of the Public Schools* (New York: Teachers College, Columbia University, 1935); H. M. Southworth and M. I. Klayman, *The School Lunch Program
and Agricultural Surplus Disposal* [Washington, DC: U.S. Department of Agriculture, 1941].

was commonly seen as a parental responsibility and concerns that the public schools would become institutions of social welfare hampered many efforts to legally sanction the provision of school meals at public expense. Even in states where such efforts led to formal legislation, these concerns shaped the language of the resulting acts.

In Wisconsin, for example, Assemblyman W. L. Smith of Milwaukee—the only major U.S. city ever to have had a socialist government—authored a bill that would permit school boards to provide lunches for children at any price, including free, so long as the amount charged did not exceed the cost of providing the lunches. The bill repeatedly failed to pass the state legislature, as numerous representatives opposed the provision of free meals for all children. When it did pass after several revisions, Governor Emanuel Philipp vetoed it, arguing that "to furnish meals at below cost, or absolutely free, is neither a sound public policy nor a public purpose, in the constitutional sense, for which taxes may be levied."[40] When a version of the original known as the Smith-Bray Bill was finally passed and signed into law in 1917, it authorized every board of education in the state to furnish lunches for schoolchildren, but it stipulated that food be served at cost and that only poor children could receive discounted or free lunches:

> The board of education of any city, however organized, or the district board of any school district may provide lunches for children attending the public schools at a price to cover the cost of the food, provided indigent children or children of poor parents may receive such lunches at such a price and under such conditions as the board of education or the district board may determine; provided, further, that the conditions under which, and the pupils to whom, such food is furnished at less than cost, shall not be disclosed to any other pupils.[41]

This bill was especially liberal in its provisions. Most states, even those that sanctioned the serving of lunches at cost to all pupils, made no special dispensation for impoverished children (Vermont was the only other state that did).[42] Although educators and health professionals across the country testified to the importance of school meals for ensuring nutritional health and educational efficiency, state legislatures either remained silent on the subject or gave their support only if the resulting programs were largely self-sustaining.

When the Chicago Board of Education requested legal advice in 1917 regarding the public financing of school foodservice, both the attorney for the board and the Illinois attorney general confirmed that there was no lawful way to spend public monies to provide meals for children directly. Faced with this clarity of legal opinion, the Board of Education searched for ways to circumvent the restrictions and remained committed to a publicly funded school lunch program. "In an exhaustive opinion rendered by the Attorney for the Board, it is held to be unlawful for the Board to appropriate money to either subsidize or directly purchase so-called penny lunches," President of the Board Edwin Davis wrote to Superintendent Shoop. "The condition, however, among the children in the schools should be relieved and I, therefore, direct you to supply penny lunches for the needed school children in the future as in the past, and I will personally guarantee an amount of five thousand dollars to be raised by public subscription."[43]

After officially commending the CSEC for their assistance in establishing and developing the penny lunch programs, in 1918 the board assumed sole stewardship of school meals in the public schools. Although the board continued to work with clubwomen and philanthropic organizations, such as the Elizabeth McCormick Memorial Fund, to provide meals free of charge to impoverished children, the board had sole oversight of financing, operations, and personnel.

Pursuant to the goal of taking full control of the city's school meal programs, the Board of Education formed a Special Committee on Health and Malnutrition of School Children in 1919 to investigate the current status of the penny lunch program and children's nutritional health. Members of the committee included Florence Vosbrink and Hilga Sethness, longtime members of the CSEC, as well as physicians and educators. The committee recommended that a "department be created for the management of the School Lunch in the Elementary, High, Normal and Special Schools, consisting of one School Lunch head or director, one assistant, one clerk, and necessary cooks and assistants." It urged that the director should have "the equivalent of a college or Normal School Education, with a knowledge of home economics, including bacteriology, hygiene and sanitation, dietetics, and the principles of cookery" as well as "experience in lunch room management, knowledge of public school administration, [and] familiarity with school problems." It also proposed "the use of the lunch as a basis for teaching a constructive program of health education and right food habits."[44] In other words, the committee pushed for a comprehensive school nutrition program, one that not only fed children but also addressed the need for nutrition education.

By the summer of 1921, the board had assumed full control of all twenty-six penny lunch programs in the city's elementary schools. This was only a small fraction of Chicago's public elementary schools (about 10 percent), but the lunchrooms operated on a self-supporting basis, with service, equipment, supplies, and the salaries of the lunchroom managers all covered by the sale of food.[45] During the 1920s, still concerned about the tenuous legality of the penny lunch programs, the Board of Education took a decidedly cautious approach. Operating the lunch programs on a self-supporting basis allowed the board to circumvent legal concerns about misappropriating public funds, but it also meant that cost—not nutritional health—defined the bottom line. The board formalized this policy in 1925, unanimously approving a set of resolutions that required "the combined costs of operation"—exclusive of equipment, space, and maintenance—to be met by receipts from the sale of food and stipulated that no foodservice expenses "be charged to educational funds without specific Board authority."[46]

Although the Chicago Board of Education remained concerned about the legality of using school funds to feed children in the public schools, it was never sued for doing so. In fact, the evidence suggests that both public opinion and legal authority tended to side with the right of school boards to operate self-sustaining meal programs for pupils. "The school lunch is no longer an experiment," declared the pediatrician and former commissioner of health W. A. Evans in his popular *Daily Tribune* health column. "The reports of teachers, physicians, nurses, and parents favor it practically without exception."[47] Public support for school foodservice had never been greater than it was in the 1920s.

In states where school boards were sued for practices connected to the operation of school meal programs, both state and federal courts invariably protected their right to do so. In these cases, the claimants were usually owners of stores or restaurants who lost business when nearby schools began serving meals. Arguments for the illegality of serving food in the schools tended to be of two types. First, it was argued that the practice violated section 1 of the Fourteenth Amendment to the U.S. Constitution, which grants equal protection under the law and due process.[48] The Fourteenth Amendment, as it was usually interpreted by the U.S. Supreme Court, prevented states from regulating or participating in commerce, except under certain limited circumstances, and protected the property of citizens from seizure and other forms of state interference. With respect to school foodservice, claimants alleged that governments were not permitted to use public monies for the operation of a business or to interfere, through direct competition, with the operation of a store or restaurant, thus depriving the owner of income (property) without due process. Second, it was argued that the operation of a cafeteria by a school board was *ultra vires*, literally "beyond the powers" conferred upon school boards by state legislatures. It was this latter argument that worried the Chicago Board of Education in particular, and it was the reason successive legal consultants advised against spending public monies to feed children in the schools.

The courts, however, tended to reject these arguments. In the 1929 case *Goodman v. School District No. 1, City and County of Denver, et al.* (32 F.2d 586), the first case regarding the legality of school cafeterias to be heard by a federal court, the Eighth Circuit Court of Appeals rejected the constitutional argument on the grounds that the school cafeterias in question were nonprofit enterprises. "The food at the cafeterias is sold at moderate prices, sufficient, however, to discharge operating expenses and provide for replacement of worn-out equipment. Profit over and above these requirements is negligible, and is not sought." The court also rejected the *ultra vires* claim:

The presumption is in favor of the proper exercise of power [by school boards], and "to enjoin such exercise it must appear that the corporation is abusing its discretion." ... It is conceded that the practice of operating cafeterias and lunchrooms in connection with public schools has been a matter of growth within the last twenty-five years, and is now almost universal, not only in Colorado, but in the larger cities of the entire country. While it is conceivable that it may be abused and carried beyond reasonable demands, there is no evidence that this has been done in the instant case.

School cafeterias were held to be lawful if conducted in good faith on a nonprofit basis for the convenience and health of the pupils.[49]

State courts handed down similar rulings. In the 1925 case *Ralph v. Orleans Parish School Board* (158 La. 659), the Louisiana Supreme Court decided that the "sale of luncheons, etc., on the school premises, during lunch hours only, to teachers and pupils only, ... is in the interest of the safe, sanitary, and efficient conduct of said schools, and that same is not an unlawful use of said buildings."[50] The Missouri Supreme Court ruled in 1925 (310 Mo. 239) that if school cafeterias were "public in character, for the public good, not for profit, and directly related to and in aid of the general and beneficent purposes of the state," their operation did not have to be explicitly mandated by the state legislature in order for school boards to be protected from liability for negligence.[51] A Texas Commission of Appeals in 1929 upheld a Houston public school statute that prohibited pupils "from taking lunch during noon recess except from [the] school cafeteria or lunch brought from home to protect [the] health of pupils." The court ruled that "it was indisputably within the power of the board to enact a rule governing the subject-matter which this rule covers, as it was designed to protect the health of the pupils during the hours they are committed to the care of the school authorities."[52] In 1931, the Texas Court of Civil Appeals similarly protected the El Paso Board of Trustees' right to operate a cafeteria and to prevent students from leaving school grounds without permission during the noon recess. "The cafeteria is a necessary convenience, and is not obnoxious to any Constitution or statutory inhibitions, and, we think, a reasonable exercise of the discretionary power conferred by law upon the board of trustees [of the public schools]."[53] In each case, the courts maintained that boards of education had the power to enact policies that protected the health of pupils and made the educational process more efficient, and that the operation of cafeterias on a nonprofit basis violated neither the Fourteenth Amendment nor state statutes.

The courts also upheld the rights of school boards to establish and enforce health requirements and employ health personnel. The first such ruling was *Hallett et al. v. Post Printing and Publishing Co.* (12 A.L.R. 919), which appeared before the Colorado Supreme Court in 1920.[54] Such rulings provided considerable support for the expanded role that schools had taken in public health. By the 1910s, medical inspection, vaccination, nursing, dental care, ophthalmology, and a number of other health services had become common in urban schools, and school boards were taking ever more responsibility for the health of children.[55] In 1914, a group of school directors in Seattle went so far as to establish a free school clinic. At its height, the clinic had nine specialty departments employing thirty-six volunteer physicians and thirteen partially compensated dentists, as well as a corps of nurses, to provide routine preventive and therapeutic care for the city's poor and working-class schoolchildren. In addition to the typical health services that many schools provided, the Seattle school clinic performed a wide range of corrective surgical procedures, including tonsillectomies, circumcisions, and hernia repair.[56]

Despite garnering support from community leaders, physicians, and the Board of Health, the Seattle clinic closed its doors in 1921. The social and political conservatism that followed the end of World War I—and the restrictive health policies implemented during the flu pandemic in 1918–1919—united parents, anti-vaccinationists, and anti-tax groups against state-sponsored health programs. When the case of *McGilvra et al. v. Seattle School District No. 1* (12 A.L.R. 913) came before the Washington Supreme Court, the state's highest legal authority ruled that the school district could not operate the clinic. This overruled the decision of the King County Superior Court, which had decided in favor of the Seattle school board. According to the opinion rendered, the clinic was "foreign to the powers to be exercised by a school district," and the court ruled further that "such power cannot be held to exist in the absence of express legislative language so providing."[57]

Courts generally made a distinction between *preventive* and *therapeutic* health care in cases related to school health services generally, but this does not seem to have been a significant issue in the legal arguments over school meals, which could be regarded as both preventive and therapeutic in the context of nutritional health. Rather, the legal issues with school meals revolved around delineation of school board powers, the extent to which the mandate to educate extended to the conservation of child health, and often vague allusion to the public good or common law.

Although the courts protected the right of school boards to operate cafeterias, all the cases that came before state and federal courts involved the *sale* of food to pupils, not the use of public monies to directly subsidize meals. As only two states (Vermont and Wisconsin) explicitly authorized the provision of food to needy children at public expense, the Chicago Board of Education had reason to question the legality of doing so in Illinois. Operating school meal programs at cost was likely not illegal, but providing subsidized meals might have been found *ultra vires* if it came before a court. Thus, in pursuing sole stewardship of school meal programs in Chicago, the Board of Education, like the school boards in most other cities, ran the meal programs at cost, charging students an amount sufficient to cover the costs of buying, preparing, and serving the food, or approximately two-thirds of the total operating costs.

The requirement that receipts cover costs, however, created a potential mismatch between the goals and the implementation of school meal programs. Since children chose their own items, and chose whether to partake at all, their tastes and preferences dictated the composition of the menus. Schools thus became economic competitors with alternate food providers, namely nearby stores, restaurants, bakeries, street vendors, and even the home. This had the potential to detract from the health goals of school meals. Speaking at the Chicago Health Education Conference, Emeline Whitcomb, a home economist at the U.S. Bureau of Education, observed: "As I travel over the country in visiting schools, . . . I so frequently find that after all that has been taught on the subject of good food habits and food selection, pupils pass the milk, vegetables and fruits on the cafeteria counter and grab for the chocolate marshmallow cakes, pickles, and sweets. They seem to like wieners and hamburgers and other similar edibles."[58] Schools had a tendency, born of legal limitations, to favor the foods that were most popular with their students, not necessarily the ones that were most nutritious or most needed by school-aged children, as those were the foods that sold. The dietitians and home economists who planned menus struggled to balance nutrition and taste, all while keeping costs sufficiently low that even the most impoverished children could partake.

In 1930, the Chicago Board of Education explicitly addressed the issue of nutritional requirements by requiring that every meal sold in the city's elementary schools "contain one hot dish, a fruit, milk or cocoa, [and] bread or crackers. A second helping of any item may be bought for an additional penny."[59] The use of categories to regulate the contents of lunches was a common solution and was ultimately included in the NSLP as the Type A and B lunches. This ensured that the meals met minimum (but not optimum) nutrition standards and supplied children with balanced meals.

At the high school level, however, students often could not return home for lunch due to the greater distances traveled; this left them fewer options and made the wares of nearby stores, restaurants, and street vendors more appealing. To protect the health of their students, some school boards used this as justification for prohibiting them from leaving school grounds during the lunch break without express parental permission. This enabled schools to offer nutritious meals without competing against the restaurants and street vendors nearby. In St. Louis, for example, despite reliance on receipts to cover the costs of food purchases and meal preparation, the menus of the city's nine public high schools included none of the foods that were popular with children but deemed unhealthful by physicians and nutritionists. "Pie, candy, popcorn, sausages, soda water, etc., are 'taboo' and are eliminated from the menus and the child receives such foods as soup, vegetables, meats, rolls, milk, cocoa, salads, and wholesome desserts." A sample menu from one of the high schools, designed by a trained

Table 1.   Sample menu from a St. Louis high school, 1925

Soup	Split Pea Soup with Crackers
Meat	Hamburger Roast with Potatoes
Fish	Baked Halibut with Creamed Potatoes
Vegetables	Egg Croquettes
	Spaghetti Italienne
Salads	Salmon
	Fruit
	Deviled Egg
	Banana and Nut
	Cheese
	Head Lettuce
Sandwiches	Minced Ham
	Sardine
	Toasted Cheese
Desserts	Snow Pudding
	Apricot Short Cake
	Fresh Fruit
	Orange Custard
	Ice Cream with Chocolate Sauce
Beverages	Bottle of Milk and a Sweet Roll
	Cocoa and a Sweet Roll
	Coffee and a Sweet Roll
	Fresh Baked Rolls with Butter

Source: Annual Report of the Board of Education of the City of St. Louis, Missouri, 1925–1926, 507.

dietitian, is shown in table 1. The lack of favorite items, such as pie, pickles, and candy, did not dampen the popularity of the lunch programs. Between 1915 and 1930, the number of St. Louis high schools with lunch programs doubled, and total sales (in unadjusted dollars) increased fourfold.[60]

By restricting the freedom of high school students to leave campus, the St. Louis Board of Education was able to control the choices of food available to those students; instead of competing with other food providers, the board restricted pupils' access to them. In doing this, the board made parents complicit in the school's health work. Since parents could grant their children permission to leave school during the lunch break, by granting that permission they absolved school authorities of responsibility for their children's nutritional health and accepted full responsibility for it themselves. This system created clear demarcations of accountability for the health of high school students.

Ironically, the very system that so successfully promoted nutritional health among St. Louis high school students was not applied to the city's elementary schools and was in fact used as an argument against doing so. In 1911, the St. Louis Board of Education had begun to develop lunch programs for younger children, serving approximately nine hundred pupils daily in five elementary schools. The menus included soup, baked beans, and stew; meat, salmon, jelly, and cheese sandwiches; bread, pudding, and gingerbread; and milk. The price of each portion averaged about 2.5 cents.[61] Unable to cover the costs of the program, though, the board abandoned the plan, noting later:

> Lunch rooms in the elementary or grade schools have never been found to be self-supporting, due mainly to the fact that the children have an hour for lunch and may go home or leave the school grounds as they choose. In such instances, the corner grocery store, the candy store or the peanut vendor has a much greater attraction than good wholesome food and the bottle of "soda pop" is the recipient of the child's nickel much oftener than the refreshing and vitalizing bottle of whole milk.[62]

The practice of returning home for lunch was quite common among elementary school pupils, who typically attended school in the vicinity of their homes. Without the power to prevent children from leaving during the lunch break—the presumption was that they returned home to eat—the board found that it could not successfully compete with the many food options that children had outside of school, and elected not to try. The city that managed one of the healthiest and most efficient high school lunch programs in the country largely ignored the nutritional health of its elementary school students. The only elementary school children in St. Louis who had access to school meals were those in the open-air schools and the school for physically disabled children, where the St. Louis Tuberculosis Society supplemented roughly one-fourth of the cost of preparing and providing the meals.[63]

The Chicago Board of Education took a different approach. Instead of compromising on participation to ensure the highest possible nutrition standards, it compromised on nutrition to ensure the highest possible participation. As early as 1923, Superintendent Shoop noted that popular foods were necessary to sustain the programs in Chicago schools:

> Suitable menus are prepared in the central office, with local variations when suitable. It is impossible to require children to follow the best meals. Managers sell sandwiches, cookies, ice cream, [and] candies as supplementary to the regular menus. Should we not do this they would be purchased from street vendors in unsanitary condition. We discourage pies and frankfurters, but serve them in limited quantities for the above reasons.[64]

In both St. Louis and Chicago, however, running the programs at cost was the bottom line; promoting health was of necessity secondary, despite the fact that health concerns had warranted the operation of school meal programs in the first place.

Indeed, under Board of Education management, Chicago developed the most extensive school meal system in the country, which by 1940 included more than sixty elementary school lunch programs and more than fifty high school lunch programs. Between the mid-1920s and mid-1930s, the number of high schools in Chicago with lunch services remained fairly constant, but the number of lunches served went up a thousandfold. The percentage of high school pupils participating also increased, from 28 percent in 1933 to 54 percent in 1940.[65]

The massive increase in the utilization of Chicago's lunchrooms during the worst years of the Depression was due as much to the success with which the schools competed with other food vendors as to the scientific planning of the menus. The official menu of the Bureau of Lunchrooms of the Chicago Public Schools, which contained all the dishes served throughout the year, included hamburgers, frankfurters, four types of pie, chocolate cake, cookies, cream puffs, seven ice cream dishes, candy bars, potato chips, and pretzels, many of which were the very elements of student diets that inspired the instigation of school meal programs in the first place.[66] Leone Pazourek, nutrition consultant for the Illinois State Department of Public Health, was shocked by the way students utilized the school lunch services: "Most of the cafeterias visited offer the pupils well-prepared foods from which an adequate lunch could be chosen, but it is appalling to see how few are choosing balanced lunches! Many of these students can glibly recite in the classroom what constitutes an adequate lunch, but their trays are evidence that the knowledge is not applied to their daily living!"[67] While Chicago's school lunches were an unqualified success with respect to the numbers of pupils served and the availability of nutritious meals, what students actually ate did not reflect the scientific management and nutritional education envisioned by reformers.

Chicago's experience of establishing and operating school meal programs exemplifies in many respects the challenges and inherent contradictions that cities faced when attempting to address the nutritional problems of schoolchildren. Despite widespread popular support for such initiatives, legal restrictions and opposition to "socialist" health and welfare programs created incentives for cities to build school meal programs that kept public costs low. This created a relationship in which school boards supplied the infrastructure and participating children bore the majority of the costs.[68] Implicitly, this sort of relationship suggests that while most people were willing to provide children the means to achieve better nutritional health, it was up to the individual children (or their families) to pay for it; those too poor to do so could rely only on private charity, not public aid. The legal, political, and social incentives led most cities to create programs that minimized costs while providing some health benefits rather than building initiatives that maximized health benefits while also controlling costs.

Yet Chicago was also unique in the extent to which the Board of Education fought for school meals and pursued a publicly funded and managed system. In most cases, school boards were permissive of such efforts but not proactive champions of them. And in some cases, as the next chapter shows, school boards actively hindered the establishment of publicly managed school meal programs.

Chapter 3

Menus for the Melting Pot

School Meals in New York City

When the Salvation Army offered free breakfasts to Manhattan children in 1905, something strange happened. Despite the grinding poverty of the Lower East Side, where the nine breakfast stations were situated, many of the children would not accept the food, and the Salvation Army eventually abandoned the effort. Lillian Wald, founder of the Henry Street Settlement House, thought the program failed "because regard seemed not to have been paid to the religious and national customs of the children, the Jewish children having felt possibly that the food was not prepared according to their ritual, the Catholics having been unable to use meat broths on Fridays, and the Italian children finding the American method of seasoning flat and tasteless."[1]

This was not the only such failure. In 1891, the New England Kitchen, begun by the nutritionists Ellen Richards and Mary Abel to improve the diets of the poor, had opened a kitchen at Hudson and King Streets in Manhattan's West Village. The installation was part soup kitchen, part educational facility, and part nutrition laboratory. Despite enthusiastic leadership, stable financing, and a desire to work with community leaders in the mostly Italian and Sicilian neighborhood, the kitchen closed after six years. The Hudson Street kitchen closed not because the menus contained foods foreign to the immigrants' palates but because the scientific approach to cooking and eating advocated by the New England Kitchen ran counter—or at least gave too little regard—to the social and cultural food traditions of the neighborhood's Italian and Sicilian immigrants.[2]

Despite these setbacks, reformers continued to pursue community-based approaches to hunger relief and nutritional improvement. A few days before Thanksgiving in 1908, the home economist Mabel Hyde Kittredge initiated a school lunch program at an elementary school in Hell's Kitchen, serving soup and bread to hungry children in the infamous Manhattan neighborhood. The following year, she founded the School Lunch Committee (SLC), a voluntary organization composed of home economists, educators, physicians, and philanthropists dedicated to improving the nutritional health and educational prospects of schoolchildren. By 1915, just seven years after the initiative began, the SLC was serving 80,000 free or low-price lunches a year to children at nearly a quarter of the elementary schools in Manhattan and the Bronx. Most of the schools were located in the city's poorest districts, and experience showed that the lunches were reaching those most in need at minimal cost to the organization. All the food served was inspected by the Health Department, and the meals were nutritionally balanced and tailored to the ethnic tastes and religious requirements of different school populations. Sparse but compelling evidence indicated that the program had reduced malnourishment among the children who partook, and teachers and principals at participating schools reported reductions in behavioral problems, dyspepsia, inattentiveness, and lethargy.

In less than a decade, the SLC had developed and implemented one of the most extensive and successful school lunch programs in the United States.[3] With the hope of expanding the service and making it a permanent function of New York City's public schools, the SLC transferred control to the Board of Education in 1919. Despite the success of the pilot program and the availability of public funding earmarked to maintain and even expand school lunch provision, the board drastically reduced meal service. What had been a carefully planned and executed school health initiative was mostly replaced by a for-profit concessionaire system with no public health or educational mandate, no nutritional requirements, no food safety inspections, no reduced-price or free meals for poor children, and virtually no over-sight of any kind.

It is overly simplistic to regard the board's abdication of a popular health, education, and social welfare program as a government agency's callous indifference to the needs of the poor. Nor was this just another instance of the discrimination against immigrants that characterized many public health interventions (or noninterventions). Although these elements were present to varying degrees, they account only for part of a far more complex issue. Because school meals were a matter of public policy in numerous domains, including health, education, labor, law, and social welfare, what the SLC regarded as a simple trans-fer from private charity to public entitlement was in fact a socially and politically charged negotiation of responsibility for children's nutri-tional health and the proper role of the public school.

Like similar grassroots organizations in other cities, the SLC hoped to demonstrate the utility of school meal programs and to convince education leaders that such programs were sustainable and valuable. Having done so, the SLC would transfer the programs to municipal control, a model of development in which the private sector experi-mented and the public sector implemented: "The function of a private organization is to experiment and demonstrate. It cannot eventuate on a large scale, and it should not if it could," argued Leonard Ayres, an education researcher at the Russell Sage Foundation and former superintendent of schools. "The function of a public organization is to eventuate on a large scale. It can seldom experiment and it lacks free-dom and flexibility in demonstration."[4] As discussed in the previous chapter, this was how school meal programs developed in Chicago, and it was a common pattern in other cities as well.

This theory of development in which private organizations devel-oped programs for broad implementation by public institutions, how-ever, presupposed clear demarcations between public and private roles and responsibilities. The growth of school lunch programs in New York City under the SLC and their reduction under the Board of Education was unusually drastic, but it reflected the uncertainty and ambiguity that existed in the quasi-official space between autono-mous private agency and public entitlement.[5] The SLC regarded meal provision as an integral part of the public school program, a community responsibility for the health and education of children. The management of such programs, for both practical and ideological reasons, rightly inhered to the city. The Board of Education, in contrast, maintained that responsibility for the feeding of children resided in the home and should not become a public burden; it was not the duty of the public schools to feed children any more than it was to house or to clothe them. The system in which private organizations developed programs that were subsequently refined and expanded by public agencies thus succeeded only when there was agreement on the delineation of responsibility for those endeavors—and on the importance of the endeavors themselves.

Numerous interests, both public and private, had a stake in the largely local school lunch debates of the early twentieth century, and the struggle over school lunches in New York City highlights just how diverse the categories "public" and "private" actually were. The Board of Education, for example, found itself at odds with the Board of Health and the Board of Aldermen, both of which supported a publicly financed school meal program. In effect, the various municipal boards represented different publics. Members of the Board of Aldermen were elected rather than appointed, and they answered to a constituency that tended to support school-based social programs. Members of the Board of Education were appointed by the mayor; they were thus more isolated (both socially and structurally) from the needs of citizens, especially the poor, and they were more susceptible to political manipulation. The private side was equally complex. The SLC, whose members included both public servants and private citizens, was a nonprofit venture that competed with profit-making restaurant owners, shopkeepers, and street peddlers for schoolchildren's patronage. The business model for school lunch programs that developed in response to legal ambiguities further blurred these distinctions.

Different municipal boards also regarded the relationship between the public and private spheres differently. To the Board of Health, the public health benefits (and resulting benefits to education) of a robust school meal program were important enough to justify bringing what had been largely a private matter—the feeding of children—under public supervision. To the Board of Education, this exceeded the purview of the public schools, and feeding children rightly remained the responsibility of the home; schoolchildren not sufficiently fed by their families could receive aid from private charity but not, as a general rule, from education funds.

This diversity of interests was only compounded by changes in education and public health administration that diminished the traditional divide between public and private. In the late nineteenth century, the germ theory of disease and the "new public health" made private spaces and behaviors the subject of public concern, for germs recognized no social boundaries.[6] As urban health authorities shifted their attention from the environment to the individual, the police powers of health departments expanded—many gained the authority to disinfect homes, confine the infectious, regulate commerce, or compel vaccination, for example—as did less formal enforcement of hygienic order, the public health equivalent of what the social theorist Jane Jacobs termed the "eyes on the street."[7] In the early twentieth century, growing concern over infant mortality and children's health had brought child-rearing, once the unquestioned domain of mothers, into the public sphere as well.[8]

This transition occurred as many states were beginning to regulate child labor and require children's attendance in school. New York passed a compulsory education law in 1874, and all states had done so by 1918. "Through compulsory attendance policies," the historian Tracy Steffes has argued, "state legislatures and local officials extended public power over children and households. They attached new regulations and intervened in decisions about children's education, health, labor, and welfare that had once been wholly private household matters."[9] After the turn of the twentieth century, schools increasingly became more than centers of education; they provided a context for the negotiation of social policy that redefined the boundaries between home and state, private rights and public welfare. The debate over school lunches in New York City offers a particularly clear example of the complexity of such negotiations, which occurred amid numerous other changes in urban public education.

This was a period of tremendous growth—and growing pains— for New York City's public schools. The first decade of the twentieth century saw school enrollments nearly double; despite a generous budget, the city could not build new schools fast enough to keep up with the expansion in population. Saddled with enormous numbers of pupils and antiquated buildings, the Board of Education initiated part-time schooling and double-occupancy classrooms in order to avoid turning children away from school. Normal operations had become extraordinarily taxing, with disastrous consequences for the quality of education. Nearly 40 percent of the city's pupils were overage for grade, and almost 16,000 fourteen-year-olds had yet to pass the sixth grade. As late as 1910, only 42 percent of all pupils completed eight years of school, many leaving to take jobs or assist their families, and the high schools lost a third of their students each year.[10]

This was the context in which school lunch programs first emerged, and from their inception, a debate ensued over the extent to which schools should assume responsibility for the health of children. An inquiry by the New York City Board of Education in 1908—the same year in which the Chicago Board of Education found that the health deficiencies of schoolchildren more than justified the need for meal provision—concluded "that there was not sufficient ground for departure from the time honored policy under which parents are expected to provide for the personal needs of their own children."[11] Yet teachers, administrators, school physicians, and social workers maintained that high rates of hunger and malnutrition were a significant impediment to health and education. School medical inspectors reported a citywide prevalence of malnourishment of approximately 3 percent, a not insignificant level of poor health, but rates as high as 40 percent were found in impoverished neighborhoods.[12] Most members of the board, however, adamantly opposed the belief that hunger and malnutrition were a significant problem and that school meals should be used to alleviate it. One referred to it as "hysterical sentimentality." Another publicly berated a district superintendent, telling her that she was "on the pay-roll of the Board of Education to do school, not settlement work."[13]

Despite the fact that numerous health and education organizations, both local and national, were promoting school meals as a useful measure against hunger and malnutrition—an increasingly visible public health concern and common explanation for schoolchildren's truancy,

inattention, behavioral problems, and poor academic performance—
the board did not regard this as something for which the schools should
take responsibility.[14] Nevertheless, meetings between members of various charitable organizations and a special committee of the Board of
Education during the summer of 1908 softened this stance somewhat,
and the board acquiesced to the installation of experimental, charitable lunch programs. That autumn, a trial lunch service was approved
under the condition that the city would incur no expenses.[15]

Principal George Chatfield of PS 51 (Forty-Fourth Street and Tenth
Avenue)—an elementary school with nearly 2,000 pupils—requested
a meal program after he found that 10 percent of his students had no
one at home during the lunch hour to feed them. With approval from
the board, PS 51 became the site of New York City's first public school
lunch program. The school was located in Hell's Kitchen, one of the
poorest and most dangerous neighborhoods in the city. It was an apt
crucible for an experimental program; if school lunches succeeded in
Hell's Kitchen, they could likely succeed anywhere.

The home economist Mabel Hyde Kittredge undertook the daunt-
ing task of running and financing the lunch program from scratch.
Only a few years earlier, Kittredge had joined Lillian Wald at the
Henry Street Settlement House. The Henry Street House, like Jane
Addams's Hull House in Chicago, helped recent immigrants and poor
residents become self-sufficient by providing educational services, job
referrals, basic medical care, and other assistance to those in need.
Kittredge founded and ran the Association of Practical Housekeeping
Centers; she created a model flat in a Russian Jewish tenement on the
Lower East Side and offered daily classes on cleaning, cooking, personal hygiene, child-rearing, budgeting, and health. The work was so
popular that she established a second model flat in an Italian district
and recruited trained, Italian-speaking instructors to run it.[16] Although
she continued this work for the next several decades, she began to
focus more and more on the nutritional needs of school-aged children.

Kittredge recruited two assistants, and they served the first lunch
at PS 51 just days before the Thanksgiving holiday in 1908. Full
meals—typically consisting of a soup, salad, or vegetable with bread,
totaling approximately 450 calories (roughly a third of a child's daily

requirement)—cost three cents, with side dishes such as crackers, fruit, and cocoa available for one cent each.[17] Kittredge attempted to cater to the tastes of the predominantly Irish children by serving soups that the children would recognize and enjoy: barley, rice and pea, and clam chowder. Although only about 10 percent of the children partook of the lunch service on any given day—the same proportion of the student body whose homes were vacant at noon—they attended regularly and filled the school's assembly hall to capacity. Kittredge responded to the interest by expanding the menu to include meat-and-potato sandwiches, baked beans, farina (corn pudding), and rice pudding, as well as sides such as prunes, bananas, apples, sweet potatoes, gingerbread, and spice cakes.[18]

For many children, this simple fare was a feast. Bill Bailey recalled the effort he expended to get food for the table as a young child in Hell's Kitchen:

> Dinner was whatever—whatever anybody would drag in. Between 38th Street and 42nd Street on Ninth Avenue was where they had all the pushcarts. . . . My job was to go up there and go underneath the pushcarts. If you could get in back of the pushcarts, you could steal anybody blind. There were always potatoes fallin' off the back and gettin' pushed out into the street. I'd go along with a little bag and pick up all this stuff. Of course, you always ran the risk of gettin' caught. I got whacked in the keester a few times, but sometimes you also picked up a nickel or penny that may have dropped.
>
> After the markets had shut down, you could help take all the pushcarts back. Many of the guys would be exhausted from standin' there all day sellin'. They'd say, "Here, take my pushcart back. Here's a penny." So I'd race like a son of a bitch down to the warehouse and run back like an idiot to look for another one.
>
> Sometimes, if there was somethin' left on the pushcart, he'd say you could take that home, too. There might be a head of cabbage, a tomato, some potatoes or rotten oranges. Whatever, it all helped. It was unbelievable, but that's what kept the family goin'.[19]

PS 51 served over 19,000 meals during the remainder of the 1908–1909 school year (approximately 200 meals per day), leading Kittredge to explore the possibility of installing the service in other schools.[20]

To expand her efforts, Kittredge founded the SLC in 1909. The committee included Principal Chatfield; Luther Gulick, director of physical training for the public schools; Margaret Poole, wife of the socialist writer Ernest Poole; and the pediatrician Ira Wile. The SLC began with three basic goals:

1. The provision of nourishing lunches on a self-supporting basis to all school children.
2. Special observation of children whose physical condition is such as to give evidence of lack of proper nourishment, in order to determine the underlying causes by a study of their homes and environment. An extension of this aim requires that these selected cases be followed up to the end that the proper agency may be apprised and appropriate action taken.
3. The formation of special classes of mothers for instruction in the proper care of children, especially in cases of poor nourishment.[21]

Kittredge wanted the school meals to be more than just supplemental feeding; she hoped to use them as a basis for broader social and public health work, especially community- and school-based health and nutrition education.

Although this program was never fully realized anywhere in the United States, the SLC had tremendous success establishing and maintaining school lunch services, which quickly became popular with parents, teachers, principals, and the children themselves. In March of 1909, the SLC began a second lunch program at PS 21 (Mott and Spring Streets), an elementary school with 2,100 pupils. PS 21 lay at the heart of Little Italy, just seven blocks north of the notorious Five Points, in an area settled largely by Genoans, Calabrians, Neapolitans, and Sicilians.

Because PS 21 had an exclusively Italian student body, the SLC employed an Italian cook and served meals congruent with Italian children's tastes. One week's menu included "minestra [minestrone] or cabbage stew, made with oil and garlic; lima beans (dried) and postu [*sic*]; rice and peas, cooked with oil or lard; lentils; cocoa and meat and potato sandwich; macaroni; and in addition each day two slices of Italian bread."[22] In developing school meal programs, the SLC embraced different cultural diets. This evoked an agenda of health promotion—getting children to eat nourishing food—over one of cultural assimilation—getting children to eat more like Americans. This aligned with national policy recommendations and common practice, which stressed working within cultural dietary practices as much as possible to improve nutrition. In Philadelphia and Boston, San Antonio and Louisville, and even in smaller cities like Bedford, Pennsylvania, early lunch programs catered to the tastes and religious requirements of the larger ethnic groups, and in no city was this more important than New York. In 1910, nearly half of the city's residents were foreign born. New York City had more Germans than Hamburg, more Jews than Warsaw, more Irish than Dublin, and more Italians than Rome, and no locality on earth had more non-natives.[23] "The one thing you shall vainly ask for in the chief city of America," noted the prominent journalist Jacob Riis, "is a distinctively American community."[24]

In addition to culturally sensitive menus, Kittredge and her associates also instituted a new payment system. Each day before school began, they sold brass lunch checks, redeemable for one meal, for three cents each. Children too poor to buy lunch could receive checks from their teachers at no charge; charitable donations collected by the SLC defrayed the cost of those meals. Thus when students lined up for lunch at noon, they each paid with an identical check, reducing the stigmatizing effects of receiving charity. Distributing lunch checks in advance also allowed the SLC to estimate demand on a day-to-day basis and communicate this to the cooks, reducing food waste and improving efficiency. Under this system, children could still purchase extra portions and sides for one cent each.

The SLC, despite its role as a charitable health and welfare organization, remained committed to a model of school meal provision based on the exchange of currency, a significant difference from the state-sponsored programs common in Europe. According to American social theory, pride would prevent even very hungry children from accepting charity. Emma Winslow, a home economist at the New York Charity Organization Society, argued that if you "deprive a person of the function of spending," then "you make that person poor indeed."[25] Even at schools without meal programs, some teachers found ways to feed needy children without hurting their pride. "The schoolteachers in P.S. 20 appointed two of us each day to clean up after their lunch in the science room," recalled a Jewish boy who grew up on the Lower East Side. "I got the point a few years later. We thought they had 'neglected' a couple of pieces of cake and two, half-full cups of coffee, but of course they wanted us to have it, without actually calling it to our attention. 'Saving face' was a big thing on the East Side."[26]

Between March and June of 1909, the SLC served nearly 9,000 lunches at PS 21 (approximately 150 meals per day).[27] Principal John Doty had nothing but praise for the program:

> In my judgment, the quality of food served . . . has been excellent. It has been well chosen to suit the taste of the children and at the same time to provide, as far as possible, the kind and quantity of nourishment needed. The improvement in dietary over that formerly provided by push carts and street peddlers has, I believe, been the cause of a distinct physical improvement in the children, and through this of a corresponding increase in mental activity.[28]

The evidence of success at PS 51 and PS 21 was not all anecdotal. Among the children diagnosed as malnourished by school physicians, 143 took lunches regularly and 81 never did; after three months, medical inspection records showed that the children eating the school lunch had gained three times as much weight on average as the children who never ate the meals.[29] Serving food was also financially viable, incurring a deficit of just $425 per school year to be supplied by charitable contributions. Kittredge theorized that an increase in attendance would make the programs self-sustaining, as the per-child cost of food and service would decrease.[30]

Yet there remained considerable need for nutritional improvement among the city's schoolchildren. Of the school children examined by the Health Department in 1910 (roughly one-third of the 600,000 enrolled pupils), nearly 5 percent were markedly malnourished.[31] In 1912, the SLC expanded to sixteen members, including the nurse and social activist Lillian Wald and Thomas Wood, professor of physical education at Columbia University. After hiring more cooks and helpers, the committee initiated lunch programs at six additional elementary schools in Manhattan, the maximum number it could manage. Three of the six schools to gain a lunch service—PS 34 and PS 92, both elementary schools with 3,700 students between them, and PS 120, a special school for boys with 120 students—were on the Lower East Side, the most densely populated slum on earth, in an area inhabited mostly by Jewish, Italian, and Eastern European immigrants. The SLC utilized the kitchen of PS 92 to prepare meals for all three schools, which were only a few blocks apart. Of the remaining three schools, PS 106 was in Little Italy, PS 107 was in an ethnically diverse, working-class neighborhood in the western part of Greenwich Village, and PS 11 was in a Chelsea neighborhood composed largely of Irish dockworkers and laborers. Superintendent of Schools William Maxwell chose the locations based partly on need—that is, schools with high numbers of malnourished or impoverished children—and partly on whether one school could serve as a central kitchen, preparing meals not only for its own students but also for those of neighboring schools, as most New York City public schools did not have kitchens.

To ensure the success of the newly established school lunch programs, the SLC focused on two issues: the dangers posed by commercial food vendors and the cultural tastes of the children. The committee chose to compete directly with the street peddlers and other purveyors of food whom students patronized during the lunch hour. Children who could not return home for lunch often bought meals from bakeries, corner stores, and lunch carts. Social workers from the Russell Sage Foundation observed that boys on the West Side often ate "at least one meal a day in the streets. . . . Crushed fruit and stale cakes and rolls are sold to children at half price, and the stalls provide candy which . . . is usually adulterated. But the boys care for quantity rather than quality."[32] Researchers from the Nutrition Lab at Teachers College, Columbia University, discovered that at one public school, children tended to buy one of four different lunches: "A tiny frankfurter and roll, costing one cent; a Swiss cheese sandwich, costing two cents; two small bananas and two long licorice 'shoestrings,' costing two cents; [or] two frosted cup cakes, costing three cents."[33] They analyzed these meals and found that the school lunches prepared by the SLC offered twice the nutritional value per penny spent.

Food safety was also a serious concern. One New York City storekeeper "advertised a keg of cider for sale at one cent a glass." When asked why the price was so low, he said the cider was so rancid that "nobody but the children would buy it."[34] Thus to "beat the pushcart man at his own game," the SLC endeavored to match the wares being offered. "When he offers tempting sugared apples on sticks, so do the schools; when he has spice cakes in fascinating shapes, spice cakes are as like as not to be found on the luncheon tables. But the school apples are good apples, the school sugar is pure sugar, the school spice cakes are nourishing spice cakes."[35] The SLC theorized that while children would tend to choose foods based on taste rather than healthfulness, careful menu planning could supply both. Once again, the anecdotal data supported the usefulness of this approach for health and education. One school had kept a medicine chest "ready for use because of the ill-effects of the push-cart diet. Since the committee had taken charge it had not been needed."[36]

In addition to competing with commercial food vendors, the SLC catered as much as possible to children's religious needs and cultural tastes, striving "always to give the children the foodstuffs of their race, but it is quite as strongly emphasized that the lunches be made up of the best and most nourishing that the nation's menu has to offer." Because the SLC's lunch programs operated largely on receipts, their success was linked to their popularity with the students. "We must constantly cater to the child's whims in order to have the lunch counter receive the three cents rather than the candy store," Kittredge observed, because "the child's taste is not always in accord with the most nourishing food at the least price."[37] The fee-for-service business model required careful planning to negotiate among children's tastes and desires, the seemingly endless varieties of cheap, ready-to-eat foods available in the vicinity of public schools, and the nutritional needs of growing children, a significant minority of whom did not get sufficient or sufficiently nourishing food at home.

By providing ethnically preferable foods, the SLC attempted to make the school lunches as attractive to the children as the foods available in their neighborhoods, even going so far as to recruit cooks from within the communities themselves. In Italian districts, only Italian cooks "who know how to cook macaroni with oil and garlic, as the children like it," were employed. When Kittredge cooked the soup one day at a predominantly Italian school, a little girl said to her, "You Americans take all the nerve out of our macaroni." Kittredge reasoned that "only an Italian can season to suit the Italian child."[38] Irish children, who would "not eat their soup thick," were served clam chowders and plain soups with bits of meat.[39] Schools in Jewish neighborhoods had Jewish cooks who prepared only kosher meals, as the kitchens were periodically inspected by a rabbi.[40] At all the schools, meat substitutes were available on Fridays in deference to Catholic tradition. The SLC promoted nutritional health by taking an approach to feeding children that was culturally oriented rather than promoting a universal diet. Although Kittredge and her colleagues utilized nutrition science in planning the menus, they did not take a completely utilitarian view of food, seeking to modify rather than supplant the diets of their mostly immigrant pupils.

Responses from the principals of all eight schools with lunch programs were uniformly positive. Word spread quickly, and administrators at eighty more elementary schools wrote the SLC requesting lunch programs of their own.[41] Because of the tremendous interest, the SLC hoped that the Board of Education would assume responsibility for the work, for the SLC lacked the resources to expand the program, could not integrate it into the larger educational mission, and had no authority to ensure that it became a permanent element of public schooling. The SLC planned to cease operations at the end of the 1912–1913 school year, "meanwhile doing all in [its] power, through a campaign in the Press and by personal appeal, to urge the Board of Education to take over the work and extend it."[42] Superintendent of Schools William Maxwell lent his support to this proposal, but the board declined to bring school meals into its official purview.[43] Although members of the board expressed support for the programs, a change in attitude from just a few years earlier, they continued to maintain that lunch programs were a charitable endeavor and not something for which the city should take responsibility. The SLC, not wanting to abandon its work, chose to continue providing meals for children in the elementary schools as it had done for the previous four years.[44]

The SLC's desire to transfer the pilot program to the Board of Education stemmed from several limitations. The committee could not integrate the lunches into the larger educational program, linking them to nutrition lessons and physical education and coordinating medical inspection, social work, and the lunch service; nor could it effect structural changes to school policy, such as banning food vendors on school grounds or preventing children from leaving school during the lunch hour without parental permission. Furthermore, the SLC had no access to public funds, which could support a much larger program and formalize state responsibility for schoolchildren's nutritional health. The Board of Education, had it decided to do so, probably could have implemented many if not all of these changes, as it was given fairly broad power over the operation of schools and the governance of education. State lawmakers, however, had enacted no legislation specifically enabling school boards to operate lunch programs using public funds, which made the issue of legality unclear.[45]

The New York City Board of Education was doubtless aware of the dubious legal status of school meal programs, which were still in their experimental stage, but popular support only grew stronger. Seeking to expand the service without the board's help, the SLC joined the New York Association for Improving the Condition of the Poor (AICP), a well-funded charitable organization working to better maternal and child health. In 1913, Elizabeth Milbank Anderson, founder of the Milbank Memorial Fund, endowed the AICP with a large trust for the purpose of expanding school lunch services. The SLC used this windfall to add lunch programs to nine additional elementary schools.[46] The committee, in consultation with Superintendent Maxwell, chose schools in the immediate vicinities of the eight with already established lunch services. Clustering the programs in this way allowed the SLC to prepare meals in four central kitchens before distribution to each school, reducing the cost of labor and equipment while continuing to serve some of the poorest neighborhoods in the city. Nevertheless, the newly expanded system required forty-five paid workers and additional labor secured through special contracts, all of whom were paid with receipts from the sale of food and the AICP's endowment.

As a part of the expansion, the SLC employed a dietitian who ensured that each dish met the criteria of the committee. The food served could not "offend religious or racial preferences," be "injurious to child development," or "fall below the Committee's standard of food value," and all meals were to be nutritionally "balanced." The SLC also worked with schools to supplement the lunch services with "parents' meetings, demonstrations, exhibits and similar activities" conducted to "bring home the practical lessons of food economy."[47] For example, Principal Harriet Tupper of PS 95 prepared charts for a Child Health Exhibit that showed how school lunches improved both attendance and classroom performance.[48] Although these supplemental activities were conducted ad hoc, the SLC hoped to elicit more community support for the school lunch movement, to increase utilization of the programs, and ultimately, to make them a permanent, publicly funded service of the city's schools.

The SLC also received assistance from the Health Department, which performed chemical and bacteriological tests on the food served to ensure its quality and safety and determined the nutritive content of different dishes.[49] This was, however, the extent of the department's involvement. "Provision should be made, both by educational methods and by some community provision," Commissioner of Health Haven Emerson wrote to Kittredge, "to make it possible for [hungry and malnourished] children to receive proper and nourishing food." While the Health Department never took a more prominent role in financing or administering the programs, it supported the efforts of the SLC and advocated for public adoption of school meals by the Board of Education.[50] Like the health departments of other municipalities, New York City's had only a tangential role in school meal programs, supporting the efforts politically and through school medical inspection and food testing but not taking a direct role in the planning or implementation of the lunch service. This was likely due in part to the Health Department's prioritization of contagious disease control and in part to jurisdictional tensions between the Board of Health and the Board of Education.[51] Although the Board of Education repeatedly declined to assume responsibility for continuing and expanding the SLC's efforts, there is no evidence that the Health Department ever attempted to do so in its place.

Just five years into the experiment, the SLC's school lunch programs were thriving. During the 1913–1914 school year, the SLC served 24,000 children 1.25 million portions of food at a deficit of less than $5,000.[52] In fact, the net deficit was only fractions of a cent—$0.00037— per portion of food.[53] The success of the programs attracted the attention of former president Theodore Roosevelt, who arrived unannounced at PS 95 on the Lower East Side to have lunch with the children. Roosevelt paid two cents for a cup of bean soup and an egg sandwich; he was so impressed with the program that he promised to work for legislation that would explicitly authorize the Board of Education to supply lunches at cost for students. (This never came to pass.) Roosevelt also noted the difference between the schools with lunch programs and those without. At one of the latter, he observed that "the children have to eat what they can get off the push carts, and it speaks volumes for their digestive powers that they don't die at once."[54]

Faced with the continued need for private funding, Superintendent Maxwell, a staunch advocate for school meal programs, lobbied the citizens of New York for donations in 1914. Some of the city's wealthiest and most prominent residents, including John D. Rockefeller, Andrew Carnegie, J. P. Morgan, and S. R. Guggenheim, as well as numerous other philanthropists, contributed a total of over $18,000 to purchase new equipment and to provide free lunches for children who could not afford to pay for them.[55] This private generosity was matched by public funding appropriated by the Board of Aldermen. In January of 1915, the Board of Aldermen issued a bond for $26,500, "the proceeds whereof to be used by the Department of Education for alterations in the equipment of public schools in the City of New York, in order to make such schools suitable for the furnishing of nourishing lunches to school children at cost." The Board of Education approved the request and estimated that the bond would be sufficient to outfit sixty schools, ten of them with central kitchens, serving 120,000 children. After the superintendent's office identified suitable sites, the bond subsequently enabled the SLC to operate lunch programs at forty-nine elementary schools in Manhattan and the Bronx. The board's Committee on Elementary Schools, however, upheld the position "that the serving of lunches by the Board of Education in school buildings is not a function of the Department of Education," arguing further "that there is no need for a universal service of lunches in the schools."[56]

In essence, the Board of Education was willing to facilitate school meal programs with money specifically allocated for the purpose—retrofitting and equipping kitchens, providing water and power—but it remained unwilling to fund them or manage them despite increased pressure from the SLC, the AICP, the Board of Aldermen, and health authorities, including the Board of Health and the New York Academy of Medicine's Committee on Public Health. Although the board resisted such pressure, it did begin to take on more responsibility in limited ways. In 1915, for example, the Board of Education managed the dispersal of the aforementioned funds. The board distributed a circular to principals, offering to subsidize the cost of providing free meals to needy children. Though warning of the dangers of pauperization, the board nonetheless offered to support the decisions of principals in distributing charity. "The principals are desired to issue free [one-cent] tickets to those who are found, after careful investigation, to be unable to pay. Free tickets should be furnished to the destitute without the knowledge of other children. Bills covering the amount of the free tickets issued should be sent to [the treasurer of the board] at the close of each week." Between January and June of 1915, more than 300,000 of the nearly 850,000 children who ate school lunches received free tickets for all or part of their meals, suggesting considerable need for the programs.[57]

Agitation from community members, health authorities, and charity organizations for the Board of Education to assume more responsibility for school meal programs intensified further during World War I. S. Josephine Baker, director of the Health Department's Bureau of Child Hygiene, argued that malnutrition rates had increased sharply as a result of rising food prices; the cost of food was more than 60 percent higher in 1917 than it had been in 1907, but wages had increased less than 20 percent in the same period. Despite extremely low rates of unemployment and numerically high salaries, many families could not afford the same amount and quality of food as they had previously.[58] Based on data from school medical inspections, the bureau estimated that while only 6 percent of children exhibited symptoms of malnutrition in 1915—double the percentage found in 1908—11 percent did in 1916, and more than 21 percent of New York's schoolchildren were malnourished in 1917. Some of this increase was an artifact of changes in diagnostic and surveillance procedures, which may have increased the rate of false-positive diagnoses, but there was no dispute that hunger and malnutrition remained a substantial children's health problem.[59] Aware of the dismal findings of the draft board medical examiners and dismayed by the poor care given children, Baker remarked that it was "six times safer to be a soldier in the trenches of France than to be born a baby in the United States."[60]

Deeply concerned about the state of children's health, both the Health Department and the New York Academy of Medicine's Public Health Committee urged the Board of Education to establish a special division for school meals and nutrition education, and to contribute public funds to the effort. Prominent health authorities, including the pediatricians Abraham Jacobi, L. Emmett Holt, and Henry Chapin, and the chairman of the Parks and Playgrounds Association, George Battle, supported making school meals a publicly funded service. The New York Federation of Labor and the Chamber of Commerce of the State of New York both endorsed a public lunch program and urged the Board of Education to support these efforts. Even the traditionally conservative *New York Times*, a Republican newspaper with distinctly anti-socialist leanings, implicitly sanctioned the proposal in a series of articles published in 1918.[61]

This widespread public pressure for greater municipal involvement ultimately convinced the Board of Education to assume responsibility for the city's school meal programs. In 1918, the SLC scaled back its lunch service to forty-four schools, maintaining programs only in the schools most in need, to facilitate the transfer of oversight to the Board of Education. To support the transition and promote expansion, the Board of Aldermen approved a $50,000 bond, available at the beginning of 1919, to create a Bureau of School Lunches in the Department of Education. The SLC considered its work to be done, having successfully demonstrated the importance and viability of school lunches, secured community support for the endeavor, and transferred management to the Board of Education, "where it logically belongs."[62] This satisfaction, however, proved premature.

Despite the large appropriation made by the Board of Aldermen for the purpose of expanding school lunch service in New York City, the Board of Education failed to act. In January of 1919, the Child Health Organization generated a report, written by the Philadelphia school lunch expert Alice Boughton, offering a plan and specific recommendations for how to utilize the $50,000.[63] After several months of inaction by the Board of Education, the Board of Aldermen adopted the following resolution:

> Whereas, the Board of Aldermen views with great concern the delay of the Board of Education in instituting in the public schools of this city a system of school lunches, which this Board on several occasions has advocated and an appropriation of $50,000 for which was made in the Budget for 1919; and
>
> Whereas, Complaints have been made to this Board that the Board of Education has unduly delayed in putting a proper school lunch system into operation.
>
> Resolved, That the Committee on General Welfare be and it is hereby instructed to arrange an immediate conference with the members of the Board of Education, with a view to securing such action as will put a proper school lunch system into operation promptly and expeditiously, and this Board further requests the Board of Education to defer action on the adoption of any school lunch plan until such conference with the Committee on General Welfare has been had.[64]

At the meeting, which included members of the Health Department and the New York Academy of Medicine's Public Health Committee as well as representatives from the SLC, Commissioner of Health Emerson "spoke of the necessity of developing school lunch work, and facetiously remarked that if the Board of Education did not see the way clear to develop it with any vision, it had better be turned over to the Board of Health."[65] Emerson's proposal, facetious or not, seems never to have been seriously considered.

A key issue was whether the Board of Estimate, the powerful board that approved the city budget, would allow the funds to cover labor costs or just the purchase of food and equipment. The Board of Education argued that the appropriation "amounted to nothing if some of the money could not be used to pay the salaries of necessary employees."[66] This was a nontrivial concern. However, the Board of Education not only failed to implement a plan to expand school meal programs; it also neglected even to maintain the programs that the SLC had already established. Between 1917 and 1919, most of the schools lost their lunch programs; only fourteen of the over sixty once operated by the SLC still remained. Instead of centralizing and expanding the school lunch program, the Board of Education abdicated responsibility and awarded foodservice contracts to concessionaires, over whom the board exercised virtually no oversight. The concessionaire system, though it may have contributed to some children's nutritional health incidentally, was little more than a profit-driven enterprise. The board established no health mandate or nutritional requirements; nor did it ensure the availability of reduced-price or free meals for poor children.

This resulted in part from major changes in city politics that adversely affected school lunch programs. After two unsuccessful attempts, Mayor John Mitchel enacted legislation in 1917 to reduce the size of the New York City Board of Education from forty-six members to seven; most major cities had already taken such a step to improve managerial efficiency. Based on the wording of the legislation, the winner of the 1917 mayoral election would also have the power to appoint all seven members, and the subsequent election of John Hylan marked the return to power—after a twelve-year hiatus—of the Tammany Hall Democratic political machine. Hylan appointed seven men to the Board of Education, none of whom had significant experience in civic or educational affairs. The new mayor exercised a heavy hand, expecting the board to be subordinate to his wishes and serve as a source of patronage; granting exclusive rights to sell lunches in city schools was a lucrative form of political capital.[67] By 1926, school lunchrooms in New York City were generating half a million dollars in business during the school year, as much as half of which went to concessionaires.[68] Instead of selling lunches to help subsidize free meals for poor children, as was common practice in nonprofit arrangements like the one established by the SLC, this was a purely commercial, for-profit model.

The Board of Education also made other changes to the school lunch service. In the few schools not ceded to concessionaires, the board made no effort to provide meals in accordance with racial or religious preferences, instead serving the same food at all schools. The menu for one week in April 1921, served in every school in Manhattan and the Bronx, was as follows:

Monday: Cocoa, buttered roll, stewed corn, stewed prunes.

Tuesday: Cream of pea soup, peanut and cottage cheese sandwich, brown Betty with lemon sauce, fruit tapioca (apricots or peaches, syrup served on top).

Wednesday: Vegetable soup, baked beans, vanilla cornstarch with chocolate sauce.

Thursday: Lima bean and tomato soup, buttered roll, cream tapioca, rice pudding.

Friday: Cocoa, salmon sandwiches, sliced fruit, and oatmeal cookies.

In addition, bread, milk, crackers, and candy could be purchased on any day.[69] Gone were the ethnic dishes of the Italians, Jews, and Irish; instead, schools citywide served a fairly bland, "American" menu containing less meat and less variety than the menus of the SLC.

This decision, the justification for which was not recorded, ran contrary to the recommendations of health and education authorities. Most organizations, both private and governmental, continued to advocate ethnically diverse menus. The U.S. Bureau of Education advised that local school authorities investigate the meal preparation techniques and food consumption habits of foreign-born populations, and suggested that "where there is a fair representation of certain nationalities among the pupils, some of their national dishes should be served at school."[70] The National Child Health Council urged that lunches be "prepared according to the tastes of the nationalities involved."[71] Even the programs developed in New York State's rural schools embraced foreign cookery: "When there are foreign-born children in the rural school, the noon lunch becomes a method for teaching them American cooking. On the other hand, the foreign-born may enrich our knowledge of cookery by teaching us their own methods of preparing food."[72] Despite the prevailing advice, New York City ceased providing meals sensitive to ethnic preferences in favor of a standardized "American" menu.

The impact of the change in menu on participation in school lunch programs is difficult to assess, as detailed participation records have not survived (or were not kept in the first place). Although the experiences of the SLC suggested that providing ethnically appropriate foods was an important element of the success of the school lunch programs, it is not clear just how important it was, and the relationship that immigrant children had with food was complex.[73]

Some immigrant children rejected American foods in preference for more familiar ones. Leonard Covello, an Italian immigrant who grew up in East Harlem, found that the "white, soft [American] bread . . . made better spitballs than eating in comparison with the substantial and solid homemade bread" to which he was accustomed. Covello attended a parochial school that the students called *La Soupa Scuola* in reference to the midday meals. Although part of the reason for sending children to the Soup School rather than the public school may have been the meals—"in those days a bowl of soup was a bowl of soup"—both the children and their parents regarded American food with suspicion. One day the school gave each student a sack of oatmeal to take home. "This food was supposed to make you big and strong. You ate it for breakfast. My father examined the stuff, tested it with his fingers. To him it was the kind of bran that was fed to pigs in Avigliano. 'What kind of school is this?' he shouted. 'They give us the food of animals to eat and send it home with our children!' "[74]

Other immigrant children rejected the foods that signaled to others their foreign origins. A desire to assimilate led them to forsake the customs and traditions of the Old World and embrace the promise and opportunity of the New World. "I avoid Italian boys and girls who try to be friendly," wrote John Fante of his childhood in New York City. "After the lunch hour I huddle over my lunch pail, for my mother doesn't wrap my sandwiches in wax paper, and she makes them too large, and the lettuce leaves protrude. Worse, the bread is homemade; not bakery bread, not 'American' bread. I make a great fuss because I can't have mayonnaise and other 'American' things."[75] Food was both a significant form of rebellion—eating that which is forbidden is a powerful way to reject tradition—and an equally significant cultural anchor, identifying the consumer with a particular religion, ethnicity, culture, or socioeconomic status.

In addition, crippling hunger may have superseded concern for dietary propriety. For example, Anzia Yezierska's semiautobiographical novel, *Bread Givers*, relates a Jewish teenager's struggle to extricate herself from the restrictive upbringing and expectations of her father, a Talmudic scholar who brought his family to New York City from Poland. After she forgoes an arranged marriage and leaves her family's home on the Lower East Side to pursue an "American" life, Sara Smolinsky's days are saturated with ever-present hunger. "Whenever I passed a restaurant or a delicatessen store, I couldn't tear my eyes away from the food in the window. Something wild in me wanted to break through the glass, snatch some of that sausage and corned-beef, and gorge myself just once." Daydreaming about food causes her to make costly mistakes at her job as an ironer in a laundry, but she cannot escape the effects of starvation. "The starvation of days and weeks began tearing and dragging down my last strength. Let me at least have one dinner with meat before I begin to starve. For that last hour of work, I saw before my eyes meat, only meat, great, big chunks of it. And I biting into the meat." She even begins to personify her stomach, the source of so much anguish. "I hated my stomach. It was like some clawing wild animal in me that I had to stop to feed always. I hated my eating. And yet I could hardly wait till my oatmeal was finished. I kept swallowing spoonfuls while it was still cooking." Sara's hunger is the most primal force in her life, and it often supplants all other considerations.[76]

While there was considerable debate about the true extent of malnourishment, and also about whether lack of food was really the primary cause, numerous New Yorkers connected their poor diets directly to poverty. For example, the boxer Sammy Aaronson, a Russian Jew who grew up on the Lower East Side, emphasized in his autobiography that

> eating was always a struggle. We ate when we had food in the house and our diet would give a social service worker the horrors. Meat soup was a big thing and we sometimes could have it once a week. Outside of that, the only hot food we ever had was potatoes. . . . Mom would send me over to the delicatessen on Hester Street where we could get a pumpernickel the size of a steering wheel for a dime. We paid a penny a herring and two took care of the whole family.[77]

Though many immigrants' lives improved after moving to the United States, poverty and hunger were still widespread. Starving children were less likely to be concerned with tradition; the laws of *kashruth* or resistance to the food served at school may have given way to sheer hunger or the desire to become more American.

Whether the abandonment of culturally sensitive menus affected the popularity of school lunch programs is impossible to say, but it likely did: as late as 1925, the Board of Education was managing only twenty-eight lunch programs (nineteen in Manhattan, seven in Brooklyn, and two in the Bronx), fewer than half the number that the SLC had run a decade earlier in Manhattan and the Bronx alone.[78] The schools used four standard menus in weekly rotation, so that every child had identical food choices on any given day. Twice as many elementary schools (fifty-three) had concessionaire-run lunch programs operating for profit, up from zero just ten years earlier.[79]

Two years later, with no indication that this situation would change, Mabel Kittredge joined with members of the city's medical, educational, and charitable organizations to found the School Lunch Inquiry Committee (SLIC). Representatives of the New York Academy of Medicine, the New York Tuberculosis and Health Association, the American Child Health Association, the Children's Welfare

Federation, the Public Education Association, the Teachers' Union, the United Parents' Association, and the Woman's City Club of New York pressured the Board of Education to change its lunch service policies. They took the board to task for leaving "the actual selection and preparation of the lunches served . . . to a business manager to decide instead of being under the complete control of a skilled dietitian."[80] The SLIC even accused the board of graft at the expense of the city's children. Not only had the number of schools with publicly funded lunch programs remained well below what the SLC had managed a decade earlier, but inspections showed "a distinct deterioration in the quality of food provided and of the equipment." Despite the increased provision in the budget for school meals—from $50,000 in 1919 to $78,000 in 1927—the city's schoolchildren were not benefiting.[81]

As a result of pressure from the SLIC and other organizations, both public and private, the Board of Education requested an additional $10,000 for the school foodservice budget and agreed to phase out concessionaires. In 1927, the board ceased to grant permits for privately operated lunch services and resolved that "concessionaires who are now operating in schools shall be shown due consideration, but as soon as practicable their services shall be discontinued."[82] During the 1928–1929 school year, the board repaired and refurbished equipment and increased the number of publicly funded programs to thirty-four, planning to add and maintain ten new programs every year if at least 20 percent of each school's pupils utilized the service. For the first time since taking over management, the board also established dietary standards: individual bottles of milk were to be available to all children; "white" bread was not to exceed 50 percent of all bread sold; at least half of the desserts had to be fruits; candy—restricted to hard candies and chocolates—had to be purchased with food; pie, tea, and coffee were prohibited; and no bottled beverages (except milk) could be sold without specific authorization from the board.[83]

Despite the Progressive ideology of private innovation spurring public incorporation, school lunches in New York City, which were tremendously successful as a private, nonprofit endeavor, fell victim to political corruption, the diversity of competing interests that shaped education and social policy, and fundamental disagreement over the balance between public and individual responsibility for children's nutritional health. Although ultimately rescued by aggressive lobbying and public demand, the city's lunch program remained less developed than those in other large cities, and it lost its distinctive characteristics, in particular the diversity of the menus and the ideology of an integrated school and community nutrition program.[84] The kind of program originally envisioned by the SLC, which combined nutrition and health education, meals, social work, community outreach, and epidemiological research, never materialized.

The limbic nature of school lunches in New York City reflected uncomfortable ambiguities in social theory, policy, and law when education intersected with public health and social justice. Reformers saw in schools the potential to reach large numbers of children, far more than charitable public health and social welfare programs could otherwise reach, but they also regarded schools as an institution that could do far more than educate America's youth. The school was an ideal site for such work, for it had extensive contact with children and parents, it was integrated into state and local bureaucracies, and it already possessed much of the necessary infrastructure. But as schools tried to provide more than education, they became a contested site in debates across a wide range of social and political issues.

Even as urban schools were radically expanding their social role—adding facilities such as playgrounds, gymnasia, and lunchrooms; expanding the curriculum to include hygiene, home economics, manual arts, and physical education, as well as special classes for disabled children; developing new programs, such as after-school sports and clubs; and incorporating new personnel, including nurses—much of this expansion, especially with respect to health programs, occurred in the liminal zone where public and private responsibilities were least clearly delineated. Just as school physicians could diagnose but typically not treat children's ailments, school boards found in most cases that they could facilitate child feeding but not fund children's food. School meal programs, in New York City and elsewhere in the United States, were thus hybrids of public and private forces, and the details of that hybridization were negotiated according to local needs and pressures.

It is important to note, however, that most of the changes in education that were occurring in the late nineteenth and early twentieth centuries were occurring in urban schools. Rural schools, prior to consolidation, saw few of these benefits, yet rural children suffered from hunger and malnutrition at rates as high as or even higher than their urban counterparts. As reformers sought to bring the benefits of school meal programs to rural schools, which the next chapter explores, they found that to do so required overcoming numerous challenges for which the well-established urban programs offered no solutions.

Chapter 4

Food for the Farm Belt

School Meals in Rural America

In the novel *To Kill a Mockingbird*, the lunch hour at a county school reveals the subtle ways in which food, health, and poverty were interconnected for many rural children.

> "Everybody who goes home to lunch hold up your hands," said Miss Caroline. . . .
>
> The town children did so, and she looked us over.
>
> "Everybody who brings his lunch put it on top of his desk."
>
> Molasses buckets appeared from nowhere, and the ceiling danced with metallic light. Miss Caroline walked up and down the rows peering and poking into lunch containers, nodding if the contents pleased her, frowning a little at others. She stopped at Walter Cunningham's desk. "Where's yours?" she asked.
>
> Walter Cunningham's face told everybody in the first grade that he had hookworms. His absence of shoes told us how he got them. People caught hookworms going barefooted in barnyards and hog wallows. If Walter had owned any shoes he would have worn them the first day of school and then discarded them until mid-winter. He did have on a clean shirt and neatly mended overalls.

"Did you forget your lunch this morning?" asked Miss Caroline.

Walter looked straight ahead. I saw a muscle jump in his skinny jaw.

"Did you forget it this morning?" asked Miss Caroline. Walter's jaw twitched again.

"Yeb'm," he finally mumbled.

Walter, the son of poor farmers, is plainly malnourished, a condition resulting from infection with hookworms and chronic underfeeding. He is three years older than Scout, the novel's narrator, who lives in town and whose father is a lawyer. Despite their age difference, Walter is smaller than Scout, his stunted growth another sign of his ill health.

Miss Caroline, the young, newly hired teacher from North Alabama—a place "full of Liquor Interests, Big Mules, steel companies, Republicans, professors, and other persons of no background"—does not yet know the children in Maycomb, the small and insular seat of Maycomb County. When Walter subsequently refuses to accept a quarter from her to buy lunch in town, Scout's explanation that "he's a Cunningham" only deepens her confusion.

> It was clear enough to the rest of us: Walter Cunningham was sitting there lying his head off. He didn't forget his lunch, he didn't have any. He had none today nor would he have any tomorrow or the next day. He had probably never seen three quarters together at the same time in his life.
>
> I tried again: "Walter's one of the Cunninghams. . . . The Cunninghams never took anything they can't pay back. . . . You're shamin' him, Miss Caroline. Walter hasn't got a quarter at home to bring you."[1]

The simple act of supervising the lunch period generates a very explicit discussion of the poor health and evident poverty of several of the children. Knowledge that was typically unspoken becomes verbalized, to Miss Caroline's great confusion and humiliation.

Walter's plight was that of many children in rural areas. The severe agricultural depression that followed World War I had plunged many into poverty, and there existed few of the charitable or medical resources common in cities.² The countryside—once symbolic of health and vitality, the antithesis of the crowded, industrial city— had fallen behind; the new standard of health was the progressive metropolis with its health department, bacteriological and chemical laboratories, municipal sanitation, clean drinking water, and hospitals equipped with the latest medical technologies.

The wretched conditions that had stimulated sanitary reform in the cities had failed to do so in the country. In most of rural America, health and medical care had changed little between 1860 and 1910. Despite the proliferation of local and county health officers after 1880, a general lack of funding and personnel led to minimal, if any, infrastructural changes. Filthy privies, antiquated housing, diseased animals, standing pools of water (an ideal breeding ground for mosquitoes), and unregulated slaughterhouses abounded, allowing common infectious diseases to persist.³

Similarly, rural schools had failed to develop along with their urban counterparts. When the National Education Association surveyed the quality of rural education at the end of the nineteenth century, it was found to be decidedly lacking. School buildings were dilapidated, teachers had minimal training if they had any at all, and supervision of school operations was lax. In addition, the legally mandated school year was often "absurdly short," as little as three months in some cases, which was compounded further by high rates of absence due to transportation challenges and the need for children to work on the farms.⁴ As late as 1913, the average number of days rural schools were in session was 138, compared with 184 in urban schools.⁵

Education, though regulated by the states, was largely a local matter. Lacking the powerful, centralized school boards and large tax revenues of cities, rural communities often built one- or two-room schools to suit their own needs. These schools supplied little more than a meeting space with rudimentary facilities—typically little more than desks, a blackboard, and a heating stove—and yet well into the twentieth century, most rural children attended such schools. During the 1922–1923 school year, for example, nearly 157,000 children in Wisconsin attended one-room country schools; 49,000 (31 percent) attended fewer than 120 days, and only 34,000 (22 percent) attended 160 days or more. At the close of the school year, there were 83 schools with a total enrollment of 1–5 pupils, 402 with 6–10, and 952 with 11–15. The majority of rural Wisconsin children attended one-room schools with fewer than 15 other pupils. Because of the extremely diffuse nature of rural education—in 1924, Wisconsin had 6,474 separate and independent school districts overseen by 19,422 school officers—there was little standardization across schools. Curricula, school buildings, supervision, and funding were largely local concerns, with substantial differences from school to school.[6]

Similar conditions existed elsewhere. In 1915, there were 3,600 residents in White County, Illinois, and 103 schools in the rural areas alone. (The county had four high schools and a number of graded town schools as well.) Townships and local boards provided little or no oversight of the schools' daily operations, and not one school in the county was able to meet the school-building standards set by the state. Health conditions were also poor. According to one survey, "The common drinking cup was to be frequently found and was usually dirty. The towel and washing facilities, if there were any at all, were dirty and insanitary. The filthy open privy was the rule. There were few exceptions." Such conditions resulted in part from decentralization, which made inspection far more difficult. In Heralds Prairie Township, there were five one-room schools despite the fact that a single, centrally located school would have been no more than two miles from any of the pupils' homes.[7]

Thomas Wood, professor of physical education at Columbia University, lamented that "the country schoolhouse is the worst, the most insanitary and inadequate type of building in the whole country, including not only buildings for human beings, but also those used for domestic animals. Rural schoolchildren are less healthy and are handicapped by more physical defects than are the children of the cities, including even the children of the slums."[8] Medical services—such as school nursing, vaccination, and medical inspection—and the teaching of health, hygiene, and physical fitness were largely absent from rural education despite their increasing inclusion in urban schools. These problems were especially pronounced in the southern states, where racial divides and widespread tenant farming maintained an enormous population of rural poor who were plagued by hookworm and pellagra, and whose cotton crops were regularly decimated by the boll weevil.

As reform-minded parents, educators, and health professionals sought to improve the nutrition of rural schoolchildren, they faced a number of unique challenges, the most significant of which was the high cost of education in rural areas. "Education costs more in money, work, and sacrifice in the country than in the city," argued the National Congress of Parents and Teachers. "The comparative isolation of farm homes and the relatively low value of property for school taxing purposes . . . mean that cooperation in the enterprise of supplying schools is more difficult."[9] When reformers confronted the growing problem of malnutrition among rural children, they did so in schools with no regular medical inspection, no play equipment, no cooking facilities, no plumbing, and often no fresh water.[10]

Although school meal programs and other public health nutrition initiatives began in the cities, by the 1910s, similar work was under way in rural areas across the country. Paradoxically, although many rural children lived on or near the farms and ranches that produced the nation's food, malnutrition rates were just as high as in the cities—and in many cases considerably higher. According to estimates made by the USDA, the average farm family produced just 40 percent of the food it consumed in 1920, down from 60 percent in 1900.[11] The shift away from subsistence farming toward commodity production—in addition to increased reliance on distributors to market crops, the high start-up cost of mechanized farming, and soaring land prices—contributed to poorer nutritional health by reducing the variety of available foods and diminishing the purchasing power of poor farmers. In fact, farmers living near cities actually had more varied diets than those living in remote areas, as they had better access to perishable foods and diverse urban markets.[12] Although the movement toward commodity production brought prosperity to many farmers (mostly to landowners in the Northeast, West, and upper Midwest), agriculture as a whole was lagging behind the rest of the U.S. economy, with disastrous effects on the health of rural children.

In response to declining nutritional health, women's groups, school clubs, parent-teacher associations, public health nurses, and others began to organize lunch programs at rural schools. They envisioned a meal service in the rural school not just as a corrective to hunger and malnutrition but as a comprehensive health plan. Ideally, the preparation of school meals would provide an opportunity to teach menu planning, dietetics, sanitary food handling, proper dish washing, safe disposal of garbage, and hand washing.[13] Because of the small size of most rural schools, lunch preparation was typically communal, involving the teacher, pupils, and sometimes parents as well. One parent noted how the lunch program at her children's rural school not only improved health and learning but also brought the community together:

> I am sure the physical condition of the children is better, especially those children who have a long way to come and have to eat breakfast so early in the morning that they will not take enough nourishment to do them with a cold lunch. The lessons which the careful teacher gives to the children in the way of table manners and proper eating are well worth the time and expense of the hot lunch. The parents also know so much better what to put up in the way of a lunch since they know it will be supplemented by some hot dish at school. The children all have to spread their home lunch on the desk before the other children, and it has made them and their mothers more careful about putting up neat and well-arranged lunches since they know the plan of all eating together. We feel the hot lunch has bound us all more closely together. The homes know more of each other and parents and teacher know each other so much better. We often hear this remark: "How did we ever get along for so many years without our little school kitchen and the hot lunch for our children?"[14]

The decentralized nature of rural schooling meant that each school determined for itself how to initiate and manage the meal service, resulting in programs that were developed in response to specific local needs. Though certain approaches proved popular, each school had a unique program.

Of the three main operational needs of a school meal program—
a food supply, labor, and food preparation infrastructure—the latter
created the biggest obstacle for rural schools. As most rural schools
had fewer than thirty pupils, the bulk purchasing of food, storage, and
transport were not a significant challenge. Students could contribute a
small fee each week to cover the costs of food or supply foodstuffs of an
equivalent value from their own farms and gardens. Rural children still
brought food from home, as even the most ambitious meal programs
were designed to supplement, rather than replace, the home-packed
lunch. Because rural schools educated small numbers of students, with
a much higher ratio of teachers to pupils than in most urban schools,
labor was also not a significant logistical problem. Unlike city pupils,
rural schoolchildren often participated directly in the planning and
preparation of meals, with tasks assigned according to age. The chief
difficulty for rural schools was finding ways to prepare meals in small,
ill-equipped buildings and raising the money to do so.

Equipping a school kitchen was often the least challenging aspect
of urban meal programs; the cost was low with respect to both the
overall budgets and the numbers of pupils served, and indoor space
was less of a problem. Rural schools, in contrast, had neither the financial resources nor in many cases the space to set up even small kitchens. (The majority of one-room schools in Wisconsin, for instance, had
from 500 to 750 square feet of floor space, which had to accommodate a heating stove, desks, a blackboard, a small library, and anything
else necessary for teaching.[15]) This led teachers and health workers to
devise a number of ingenious solutions.

Nellie Farnsworth, a home economist from South Dakota, suggested that rural communities could obtain equipment for preparing
meals at school with minimal expense. The equipment "needed for
preparing one warm dish at school" was not very expensive (assuming
that the children could bring their own utensils, plates, and drinking
cups) and was readily available (see table 2).[16] Although $11.50 was
not a lot of money even in 1916, neither was it insubstantial; that was
nine days' wages for the average farm laborer.[17]

To obtain these items, teachers and parents conceived several different plans. Although many school boards could and did supply such

Table 4.1.   Sample list of equipment needed to operate a school lunch service in a
rural school, 1916

Quantity	Item	Cost
1	Two-burner blue flame oil stove	$3.25
1	Portable oven	$3.25
1	Frying pan	$0.40
2	Granite kettles	$0.80
1	Sieve	$0.10
2	Aluminum tablespoons	$0.20
2	Aluminum teaspoons	$0.10
1	Steel knife	$0.10
2	Asbestos mats	$0.10
2	Granite basins	$0.40
1	Dover egg beater	$0.25
1	Dish pan	$0.50
1	Draining pan	$0.30
1	Two-quart double boiler	$1.75
Total		**$11.50**

Source: Nellie Wing Farnsworth, *The Rural School Lunch* (St. Paul, MN: Webb, 1916), 7.

equipment, rural boards were less likely to support such initiatives than urban boards, due both to the shortage of funds and to the general conservatism of rural board members.[18] Country teachers often had to raise money or secure equipment themselves. One Minnesota teacher held a shower to gather the necessary items; she invited "all mothers and women interested in the school" to a social, requesting that each bring with her one of the things that she had designated at the local store. This not only generated all the needed equipment (plus additional supplies) but also acquainted the residents of the area with the plan to prepare meals in the school.[19] Other schools held health pageants or put on health plays to raise money and stimulate community interest in the needs of children.[20] In New Hope, Wisconsin, one school used district funds to buy an oil stove and money raised from school socials to purchase cooking utensils; the combination of public and private funding made it possible to begin a hot lunch program.[21]

Another home economist in South Dakota suggested accumulating in stages the equipment needed to prepare meals at school. During the first stage, a school required only a stew pan with cover, a large stirring spoon, a dishpan, and some towels. Students would bring their own utensils, plates, and cups, and cooking could be accomplished by using the heating stove. This minimized the investment in equipment but made possible the preparation of simple dishes. If this initial stage aroused the interest of parents or the school board, then more equipment could be purchased, such as an oil or gas stove, an oven, a double boiler, a skillet, and utensils.[22] Endeavors such as these equipped numerous rural schools with rudimentary infrastructure for food preparation.

Some schools even managed a modest meal program with virtually no equipment. In Sullivan County, a remote region of northeastern Tennessee, Betty Stuart, "a quaint mountain woman," began a hot meal program at the request of the county supervisor. When she arrived at the Harr School in the early 1920s, there was no stove, so she built a stone oven outside the school. Every day each child brought a bowl, a spoon, and bread, along with "a handful of dried beans." Stuart washed the beans and let them cook on the outdoor stove during the morning lessons, serving them to the students at their desks. Each child washed the bowl and spoon at home, as the school had no running water.[23]

In colder parts of the country, schools typically had a heating stove, which could be used for cooking as well. Repurposing heating stoves for cooking, however, presented a number of difficulties. Although it cut costs by combining functions, there were several technical challenges. The typical unjacketed heating stove, used in most rural schools until the 1920s and still common in the 1930s, had no horizontal surface on which to cook. Furthermore, heating stoves were often small, leaving little space on top for use, and the temperature was not readily adjustable.

Despite these shortcomings, rural teachers, parents, and extension workers devised several strategies. One circular suggested baking potatoes in the ash pan of the stove, a practice that did not require a cooking surface or additional equipment.[24] A Pennsylvania girl remembered that at her school, the pupils would always "bring in potatoes and put them in an hour or so before lunchtime."[25] In Elkhart County, Indiana, baked potatoes were the most commonly prepared food in one- and two-room schools.[26] Another pamphlet explained that a teacher could cook a casserole in a jacketed stove by placing it in the space between the door and the fire box.[27] A teacher in Minnesota had one of the boys "make a stout wire frame to fit over the top of the stove which was round and would not hold a kettle." This made it possible "to serve a soup, cereal or chowder every day during the entire winter term."[28] While such innovations were not limited to rural schools—the high schools in Rochester, New York, for example, cooked food by diverting the waste steam from the heating plant to the kitchen, eliminating the cost of cooking fuel—they were often the only way to provide students with warm meals in remote locations.[29]

Not all reformers, however, saw the reappropriation of heating stoves for cooking as a good thing. "In a number of schools the hot lunch has been prepared over the school heater, the only extra equipment being a large kettle, a spoon, and a measuring cup," an extension worker from Illinois wrote. "If it were a question of feeding the stock, the necessary $25 or $30 for a good kerosene stove, double boiler, and other utensils would be spent without question."[30] Moreover, not all innovations to overcome shortages of money and space were successful. In one district, a mothers' club decided that each member should take turns preparing a noon meal for the schoolchildren. The mothers would purchase the food, cook it at home, and then bring it to the school to be served.

> For a time this seemed to work very well. There was no expense to the district . . . [and] no extra work for the teacher. The children liked it. It was quoted in various school journals as a very successful method. Gradually, however, comparisons of the meals created rivalry between the women. The school lunch became a contest in cookery and with this the expense of providing it became almost prohibitive. The women who felt that they could not afford to serve a banquet to the school children, refused to have their children so fed. As a result, a feeling of bitter resentment arose in the neighborhood. The school, instead of being the one community interest, became the cause for community quarrels. It will require considerable tact to interest those people again in a hot school lunch.[31]

Failures such as this were not common, but rural areas were particularly dependent on direct community cooperation and investment. Even when school boards offered financial assistance, teachers and parents—and often older students—had to plan and organize the programs, provide all or most of the labor, purchase the food, and do any necessary accounting. For example, home economists at the Massachusetts Agricultural Experiment Station found that 80 percent of the state's rural school lunch programs were "both sponsored and managed by the teachers, with no help except that of their pupils."[32]

Although there remained a need for direct community involvement, several technological innovations made the rural lunch at least feasible for many schools. The fireless cooker, for example, allowed teachers to serve a warm dish during the lunch break without doing any cooking during class time. The fireless cooker, which could be purchased or made, consisted of a pot tightly nestled within an insulated container. To use it, one would prepare a stew, cereal, or other similar dish in the inner pot, bring it to boiling on a stove, and then place it within the insulated container, where it would continue to cook for the next several hours. At lunchtime, then, the teacher could simply remove the lids and serve a hot, fully cooked dish. The fireless cooker not only solved the problem of cooking in a small school but was cheap and easy to make. In Douglas County, Minnesota, the teachers and pupils at two rural schools constructed fireless cookers from "candy pails, asbestos, tin pail[s] and hay."[33]

The most popular innovation that allowed rural schools to serve meals to pupils was known as the "pint-jar method" or the "Wisconsin method." Jeannette Pugh, a public health nurse employed by the Wisconsin State Board of Health, developed the idea around 1920. In the course of providing health services to rural schoolchildren, she found that only 22 of the 125 schools in her territory had meal programs for the pupils. The desire was present, but the means were not. Pugh commissioned a tinsmith to make a wash boiler in which rested a removable rack with thirty-two holes, each sized to hold half-pint jars, which were widely used to preserve fruits and vegetables. Dishes such as soups, stews, cereals, and cocoa could be distributed among the jars and placed in the rack. Thirty to sixty minutes before the lunch break, the teacher simply had to pour a little water in the boiler, put the lid on it, and place it on the stove. At the noon recess, the teacher then distributed the jars, and the children had a warm dish to eat.[34]

The pint-jar method held a number of advantages for rural schools. Besides requiring little labor, minimal equipment, and only a small monetary investment (if any), it solved a number of problems facing one-room schools. First, it was a method that not only enabled the serving of communal dishes but also allowed pupils to bring their own pint jars, filled with food prepared at home, to be heated at school. This was especially helpful in areas where winter temperatures dropped below freezing. A midwestern schoolboy described in poetic detail the consumption in winter of half-frozen lunches: "Our dinner pails (stored in the entry way) were often frozen solid and it was necessary to thaw out our mince pie as well as our bread and butter by putting it on the stove. I recall, vividly, gnawing, dog-like, at the mollified outside of a doughnut while still its frosty heart made my teeth ache."[35] After the introduction of the pint-jar method, instead of the usual contents of the lunch pail—"cold pancakes, salt pork, cold potatoes, pie and bottles of cold tea or coffee"—children could have warm, appetizing dishes during the noon recess.[36]

Second, the pint-jar method required no food preparation or cooking to take place at the school. This not only benefited schools with minimal space or no access to cooking equipment, but it also took no time away from teaching. The local teacher or parents' group could prepare a dish at home and then simply bring it to the school to be heated and served. For teachers in one-room schools, most of whom were young and inexperienced, the pint-jar method reduced the labor burden.[37]

Lastly, the pint-jar method was ideal for schools with no source of water. The teacher had only to bring water enough for the boiler; the children could each take home their own jars to be cleaned and refilled, so that no dishwashing need occur at the school. While the lack of drinking water remained a challenge, the pint-jar method could at least reduce the amount of water that needed to be hauled to the school.

Because of its convenience, low cost, universal applicability, and ease of implementation, the pint-jar method proved enormously popular. In one Colorado district, the mothers each prepared food for their own children but agreed to use the pint-jar method in order to ensure that the children ate a hot, nourishing meal at school.[38] Elma Rood, director of health education in Mansfield, Ohio, found a similar situation when she visited rural schools in her area. "I will tell you some of the things that were in those jars," Rood wrote. "There was a jar of tomato soup, one cream of tapioca, six rice with meat cooked in it, one jar of cocoa, one of beans. There were a variety of other things but I noticed that the lunches were all very nutritious."[39]

After the pint-jar method was introduced to West Virginia in the early 1920s, women's clubs and parent-teacher associations sponsored programs "because the idea of providing hot lunches for children was popular."[40] Pupils also responded positively to the pint-jar method. One Wisconsin resident recalled that "in the winter, lunch often included a pint jar of soup or chili. A pan of water always steamed on the top of the stove, for the purpose of adding humidity to the always too dry room. Those with soup jars placed them in the pan of water during morning recess, and by noon time the soup was warm and deliciously ready to eat."[41]

However, when it came to addressing the lack of space and equipment in small rural schools, one suggestion was conspicuously absent. Despite the technical difficulties associated with cooking, no home economist, extension worker, or public health nurse suggested instead that schools prepare exclusively cold (uncooked) dishes such as sandwiches or canned fruits and vegetables. The overwhelming preference for hot food was in part a practical consideration. In rural areas, children typically attended school during the coldest months of the year, when they had the least amount of work at home. During the winter months it was more important to provide warm food, and even cold food often had to be thawed prior to consumption. However, most nutritionists and physicians argued that hot food was important year-round. A pamphlet distributed by the Pennsylvania State Department of Public Instruction, for example, claimed that warm food "saves the body heat and energy, gives a feeling of comfort and warmth, and assists digestion in a general way."[42]

In fact, school meal promoters in rural areas were far more vocal about the necessity of a *hot* meal than were their urban counterparts. The county nurse in Price County, Wisconsin, for example, told parents and teachers that "better digestion is incited by the hot food," which would produce better schoolwork, better health (especially decreased malnutrition and tuberculosis), better table manners, and better food choices. She also recommended that schools without funding or adequate equipment begin with the simplest of hot dishes. "In the beginning it is advisable to only serve a cup of hot milk, hot cocoa or soup. The equipment needed for this is very simple and inexpensive. Later more equipment may be added."[43] Even the language reflected this distinction; while cities often employed the term "penny lunch," even in cases where the cost of a meal was more than one cent, rural areas typically used the term "hot lunch." Low cost was a key selling point for school meal programs in many urban areas, whereas the warmth of the meal was the defining characteristic in country schools.

The recommendation of warm lunches also aligned with physiological theory. Physicians and nutritionists frequently described cold meals as indigestible or even unhealthful; hot meals, in contrast, were the exact opposite. "Hundreds of cold meals in the course of the eight years in school," argued one nutritionist, "may mean the difference between a poorly nourished child and a well-nourished child; poor health and good health; poor digestion and good digestion."[44] As late as 1943, the food distribution administrator for the federal government claimed that "it is fundamentally true that hot lunches served at school are far more nourishing than cold meals brought from home."[45] Medical texts generally confirmed this view, but belief in the benefits of warm meals bordered on the metaphysical; advocates of school meals appealed less to scientific knowledge than to the intrinsic goodness or wholesomeness of warm food.

Although the ingenuity of teachers and health workers helped to overcome the difficulties of preparing and cooking food in schools with limited space and facilities, the development of school meal programs in rural areas was usually sluggish at best. The decentralized nature of rural schooling, geographic isolation, the conservatism of many school boards, and a lack of financial resources slowed the development of systematic school meal programs.

Several developments in the late 1910s and 1920s, however, helped expand nutrition work in rural schools. During this time, state boards of health began to provide health services to rural communities, typically through a network of visiting or community public health nurses and county boards of health. Ideally, county boards were to be staffed by a full-time health officer, a nurse, a sanitary inspector, and a clerk, but in reality, they often had only one or two of those positions. Nonetheless, county boards delivered basic health services to numerous communities that had never had contact with public health infrastructure of any kind. Extension services, operated by land-grant universities and agricultural colleges, sent medical and scientific experts to offer continuing education classes for adults and basic assistance in setting up and running school meal programs, nutrition classes, well-baby clinics, and other health initiatives.

At the turn of the twentieth century, most state boards of health were underfunded, understaffed—largely by volunteers—and basically ineffective. When the Rockefeller Sanitary Commission, a privately funded health initiative, announced in 1910 that up to 40 percent of southerners were infected with hookworms, it energized rural public health development. In the next decade, the U.S. Public Health Service took an active interest in pellagra, typhoid fever, and malaria, all of which were predominantly rural problems by that time. The influenza pandemic of 1919 and the Mississippi Valley floods of 1927 also stimulated public health efforts in rural areas. The U.S. Children's Bureau, the National Tuberculosis Association, the Milbank Memorial Fund, the Commonwealth Fund, and the American Red Cross for the first time sponsored rural health programs, and many sent public health nurses to rural areas. In addition, county health departments began to provide basic health services such as nursing, health education, disease surveillance, and vaccination.

The USDA also began to take an interest in issues of rural health and nutrition. When President Abraham Lincoln signed the Act to Establish a Department of Agriculture in 1862, the newly created department had no stated public health function, but part of its mission was "to acquire and diffuse among the people of the United States useful information on subjects connected with agriculture in the most general and comprehensive sense of that word."[46] With this broad, vaguely defined assignment, the USDA had exceptional freedom to determine its own functions. In 1888, Commissioner of Agriculture Norman Colman argued for the inclusion of food and nutrition research in the department's activities:

> The chief agricultural product is food, which all need. More than half of the earnings of the working people in this country . . . must be spent for food, and yet even the most intelligent know less about the relation existing between the nutritive value and the cost of their food than about the value as compared with the cost of their clothing, houses, fuel, or any of the other necessities of life. This lack of popular understanding of the pecuniary economy of food, and of its physiological economy as well, results in great loss of money and injury to health. For improvement the first requisite is information, that which comes only from research. . . . I venture to suggest that inquiries in these directions are appropriate for this Department.[47]

In 1894, Congress appropriated $10,000 "to enable the Secretary of Agriculture to investigate and report upon the nutritive value of the various articles and commodities used for human food, with special suggestion of full, wholesome, and edible rations less wasteful and more economical than those in common use."[48] This marked the first time that the federal government granted money exclusively for the study of, and distribution of information on, human nutrition, and by the turn of the century the appropriation had doubled. The work was to include investigations of the nutritive contributions of foods, the process of digestion, the composition of dietaries, and publication of the results for both lay and professional audiences.

Further legislation only deepened the USDA's public health responsibilities. The Hatch Experiment Station Act (1887), the Smith-Lever Extension Service Act (1914), and the Smith-Hughes National Vocational Education Act (1917) created a close relationship between the USDA and state governments regarding agricultural research and education. The Hatch Act provided $15,000 annually to each state for the establishment and maintenance of agricultural experiment stations "to conduct original researches or verify experiments" on subjects of agricultural importance as determined by the state.[49] Most of the USDA employees had come from the land-grant colleges that hosted the experiment stations, creating tacit relationships between the federal government and local colleges, but the Hatch Act made these relationships more formal by tasking the USDA with coordinating research and public education efforts among the states.

Similarly, the Smith-Lever Act provided $10,000 plus additional matching funds to the states for the establishment or maintenance of rural extension services. Extension workers established programs and provided adult continuing education in agriculture, nutrition, health, child-rearing, and many other topics. The federal government thus provided the states with funding for health education and research, and the USDA coordinated these efforts.

The Smith-Hughes Act provided federal funds for vocational education and teacher training. The language of the act classed home economics—a significant component of which was the study of foods and nutrition—as vocational, and thus provided funds for the training of teachers in a variety of nutrition topics, including how to begin and operate a school meal program.

Collectively, this legislation provided resources to the states that could be used to promote school lunch initiatives in rural areas. The effects of this attention to rural health needs was particularly strong in Wisconsin, where the combination of federal and state legislation, along with the initiative of extension workers and public health nurses, facilitated particularly high rates of rural school meal service.[50] When Governor Emanuel Philipp signed the Smith-Bray Bill into law in 1917, authorizing all boards of education in the state of Wisconsin to serve meals to pupils at cost—or below cost to those who could not otherwise afford them—it was the first such law passed in the United States.[51] The Smith-Bray Bill removed any legal impediments to providing meals for schoolchildren at public expense, a particular boon to rural children who had little or no contact with the charities that supported such programs in cities.

In this same period, public health services came to many parts of rural Wisconsin for the first time. The organization of county health departments began in 1911, and both the State Board of Health and private health organizations began to take an interest in rural areas.

For example, in 1916, Wisconsin had 125 public health nurses, only 9 of whom worked outside of the cities; by 1923, the state had 288, with most of the expansion occurring in rural areas.[52]

All of these factors made possible an ambitious project to promote school meals in rural Wisconsin. In 1919, at the beginning of a severe agricultural depression, two University of Wisconsin extension workers, Nellie Jones and Gladys Stillman, launched a statewide campaign to introduce meal programs to rural schools. In doing so, they facilitated one of the largest expansions in rural school foodservice in the country. Just three years after they commenced their work, nearly half of the rural schools in Wisconsin were operating a school meal program.

Nellie Kedzie Jones was a pioneer in the field of home economics. In 1887, she became the first female professor at Kansas State Agricultural College, where she earned both a bachelor's and a master's degree, and she was also the first woman to head a department there. After lobbying the state legislature, she secured funding to build Domestic Science Hall, the first structure built specifically for home economics at an American university. After stints at several other colleges, Jones settled in Wisconsin. Between 1912 and 1916, she had a regular column in the *Country Gentleman* magazine, in which she advised rural women on topics in housekeeping, cooking, and child-rearing. In 1918, Jones became Home Economics Extension leader at the University of Wisconsin College of Agriculture, a position she retained until 1933. In her official capacity, she traveled throughout the state, speaking to women's clubs, granges, homemakers' clubs, and groups organized by county demonstration agents.[53]

Gladys "Sally" Stillman received her BA and MA in home economics from the University of Chicago. She subsequently served as food and nutrition specialist in the University of Wisconsin College of Agriculture's Extension Service from 1919 until 1953, writing and lecturing on topics in food and nutrition. Her pamphlet "The Hot Lunch in the Rural Schools" went through four editions, and the Extension Service distributed more than 40,000 copies of the first edition alone.[54]

One of the first projects Stillman proposed when she began her work in the Extension Service was to establish hot lunch programs in rural Wisconsin schools. Her ultimate goal was to improve the health of rural children by increasing milk consumption, serving children "such dishes as to make balanced lunches," and teaching them "to like simple, wholesome foods." Stillman noted in her proposal that there were no legal impediments to the work she proposed. Her highly detailed and carefully devised plan involved a number of steps. Stillman decided first to survey the counties, choosing two or three in which to begin work, and then to "select ten or twelve schools in each county where the teachers will cooperate and where the lunch seems needed." After identifying suitable schools, she would meet with the teachers, demonstrate the planning and conduct of a hot lunch service, and designate a "community leader"—often a teacher, county nurse, or local home demonstration agent—to take responsibility for continuing the work. Stillman suggested that the community leader maintain regular correspondence with the teachers and the Extension Service once the lunch programs were operational and that newsletters and newspaper articles be published reporting the goals, implementation, and results of the work.[55]

With Jones's support and guidance, Stillman began to give lectures and demonstrations on how to start a hot lunch program in November of 1919. By the following June, she had visited seven counties—Barron, La Fayette, Lincoln, Portage, Rock, Shawano, and Winnebago—and helped to establish permanent school meal programs in five of them. Her visits often had immediate results: "In November at the request of the county nurse from Barron County, I spent a week with her visiting schools and demonstrating the hot dish at noon. . . . We visited eight schools, five of which continued the hot dish throughout the winter months and reported to me of their success in the work." The Colonization Company in Lincoln County offered to donate half of the money for necessary equipment to any school that could raise the other half; after Stillman demonstrated how to prepare a hot lunch in eleven schools, eight of them took the offer. In addition to these activities, Stillman lectured at several county normal schools, which prepared teachers to teach in one-room schools, urging them to emphasize the importance of rural school meal programs in their curricula. She also initiated a rural teachers' training class to help teachers learn how to begin and maintain a school meal program.[56]

The hot lunch idea took off immediately in Shawano County, which had about 10,000 school-aged children and 105 rural school districts. Prior to 1920, the school inspection cards used by the County Superintendent's Office had no place to indicate whether a hot lunch was provided. In the 1920–1921 school year, following Stillman's visit, Gertrude Ainsworth, a supervising teacher, inspected nearly 100 rural schools; 42 had no hot lunch service, 33 did, and 15 were planning to start one. Half the rural schools in Shawano County had either initiated a lunch program or were about to do so. In a number of the schools that did not have lunch programs, Ainsworth noted that "warm lunches should be served" or that they "could easily be arranged for."[57] While it is not clear if this expansion was a direct result of Stillman's lecture, the timing is suggestive. The county superintendent of education noted that "the advantages [of a hot lunch] rank with ventilation in importance. In one case we are taking precautions against nasal, throat, and tubercular troubles and in the other, against dyspepsia and allied ailments. If a warm, midday meal is desirable for the adult at home, it would seem to be equally so for the growing child at school."[58]

Stillman's work proved tremendously successful. In the 1918–1919 school year, before she began her campaign, just 215 of the roughly 6,500 rural schools in Wisconsin served a hot dish to pupils. The following year, 1,551 did so. By the 1920–1921 school year, 3,148 rural schools, nearly half the rural schools in the state, reported that the service of at least one hot dish daily was part of their health program.[59] To put this in perspective, only 346 rural Illinois schools served a hot dish or meal in 1921, even though Illinois had a rural population of 2.1 million people while Wisconsin had a rural population of only 1.4 million.[60]

The reports of Stillman's appointed community leaders showed improvements in both health and school work at the schools where hot lunches were introduced. Of the thirty-three reports submitted in 1920–1921, "one third showed the children had better health and made better gains in weight while one reported fewer colds in the school as a result of the work. One half of the reports indicated better [school] work and more interest in the work by the children. One third reported more fruit and less pastry brought by the children in the lunches from their home[s]." The children themselves responded positively as well. "I am glad you came to our school," twelve-year-old Mildred Riley, a pupil at one of the schools to receive a hot lunch demonstration, wrote to Stillman. "We are having hot lunches every day now, and they taste fine with cold sandwiches."[61]

The Extension Service also implemented educational campaigns of a more theatrical nature. In addition to giving lectures and doing demonstration work, Stillman and other nutrition specialists designed contests for schoolchildren. They challenged contestants to create posters or booklets that promoted milk drinking, hot lunches in the schools, or vegetable consumption; the winners received prizes and saw their work displayed at fairs and reproduced in pamphlets. Thousands of Wisconsin children entered their work in 1920, and the contest was repeated in subsequent years.

During a weeklong campaign in 1921, the Extension Service enlisted a store across from the state capitol—where rural representatives would presumably pass by—to demonstrate the composition of proper lunches and encourage children to drink milk. Four children sat at a table in the store's window display, drinking milk and eating a nutritionally balanced meal, while signs and posters explained the benefits of doing so.

Having built up a sizable interest in rural school meal programs across the state, Stillman began to focus on other endeavors. Although she continued to promote hot lunches, she did so in the context of more general nutrition work, and not as a special project. "It seemed wise not to put any special time on this project for the year 1922–1923," Stillman wrote in her annual report, "but to include talks and encourage the rural hot lunch whenever possible."[62] This was due in large part to the success that she had in making meal programs an integral part of rural schooling. Throughout the 1920s, nearly half of Wisconsin's rural and state graded schools maintained a meal program for students. Even during the Great Depression, far more rural schools served hot dishes to students than had before Stillman began her work in 1919.

The school meal promotion efforts that Jones and Stillman initiated spread well beyond the counties in which Stillman was most active. For example, starting in the fall of 1919, the Sauk County schools began to develop public health nutrition programs. The county superintendent, A. H. Martin, encouraged all schools to weigh and measure children monthly, "initiate the use of the hot lunch or the serving of milk," and provide extra milk for the underweight when possible. "If a hot lunch is served during the noon hour," Martin proposed, "the menu should be determined by the morning and evening meal of the children who are anemic and underweight. One hot dish as soup, cocoa, vegetables, pudding or a cereal may be served."[63] Martin envisioned the school meal program, as did most other advocates, as part of a larger system of health and social services, combining education, social work, medical care, and nutritional support.

One of the core nutrition education goals that most schools had was to reduce the consumption of coffee and tea among children.[64] When the Sauk County nurse, Palma Ghran, visited the Man Mound School in the winter of 1920, she found that none of the school's sixteen children consumed coffee, a relative rarity. Asked why they refrained, many replied that "it is not good for you," but she found other explanations quite shocking:

> Coffee is a deadly poison.
> It will make you black.
> It will make your teeth come out.[65]

The *Sauk County Schools*, a monthly publication prepared by the county superintendent, urged teachers to correct these misconceptions by explaining the chemical nature of coffee and tea and the physiology of growth. It was important, the superintendent emphasized, not just that children did the right things but that they understood why.

The state superintendent of education also promoted school meal instruction in county normal schools. "Warm lunch work is necessarily taught in county training schools," wrote the state superintendent in 1922, because there was an expectation that teachers in one-room schools should be prepared to institute and manage such programs.[66] The state superintendent had stated this explicitly in a letter to two Door County superintendents in 1921: "Preparation of these lunches would afford excellent practice for the students who are later to manage such lunches in the country schools."[67]

By the late 1920s, the state superintendent had developed boilerplate language promoting warm school meals that was included in communications to county superintendents.

> It is very desirable for the health of the children that a warm dish be served in every rural school through the school year. The pint jar method has been found to be the simplest and perhaps the most satisfactory method to use in providing this warm dish. We find in many schools very fine control of the lunch period. Much should be done to train children to proper lunch habits in every way.[68]

This exact language was included in letters to superintendents of Barron, Bayfield, Burnett, Dane, Grant, La Fayette, and Vernon Counties, and likely in many other communications as well. Inspections of rural schools also began to include information about school meal provision. For example, one noted that schools in Portage should "try to arrange for fresh drinking water to be used by pupils at least three times during the school day. A definite program for the conduct of the noon lunch period would be very desirable."[69] Like the boilerplate language quoted above, variations on this theme were included in numerous inspection reports submitted to the state superintendent.

While it is impossible to know much about how most rural lunch programs were actually conducted, it is clear that by the 1920s, substantial efforts were expended in Wisconsin and in many other states to promote rural school meals. Although these programs were not as comprehensive as those developed in cities—at best, most rural schools could provide only one simple dish and not a complete meal— a remarkable level of ingenuity went into making that possible. Most one-room rural schools had none of the administrative, financial, or infrastructural resources of city schools. Nevertheless, many country schools found ways to operate a regular meal program. In Wisconsin, a combination of state legislation, improved access to basic public health services, technical ingenuity, and aggressive promotion and education made possible a tenfold increase in the rural schools with warm lunch services. Most states did not experience such dramatic improvements, but many did significantly expand rural school meal provision through their extension services, state and county health departments, and public education campaigns.

During the 1930s, one-room schools were increasingly consolidated into graded schools, with bus services to transport children living long distances from the new facilities. As rural schools became more like urban schools, rural meal programs became more like urban ones, with plate lunches, a greater selection and variety of foods, and centralized management, financing, and oversight. When the Great Depression hit rural areas, which had already been suffering through an agricultural depression since the end of World War I, New Deal legislation made it possible not only to sustain many rural meal programs but even to expand them. With the federal government taking a more direct role in school foodservice nationwide, local school meal programs soon became the subject of national politics.

Chapter 5

"A Nation Ill-Housed, Ill-Clad, Ill-Nourished"

School Meals under Federal Relief Programs

When the stock market crashed in October of 1929, it did not so much cause the Great Depression as herald its arrival. The agricultural economy was already badly depressed.[1] High tariffs and interest rates, currency instability, and declining consumption in the late 1920s all contributed to a national economic slowdown, but it was the years between 1929 and 1933 that witnessed the worst of the decline: real GNP fell by 30 percent, new investments failed to keep pace with the depreciation of existing stocks, national income was cut in half, and nearly one in four Americans failed to secure gainful employment. Of those lucky enough to have work, almost three-quarters toiled only part-time. U.S. Steel, which employed 225,000 full-time workers in 1929, employed no full-time workers in 1933, and production decreased 81 percent. The American Locomotive Company manufactured only a single engine in 1932 after averaging six hundred per year during the 1920s. Banks had foreclosed on almost a million farms by 1932, and income from agriculture was less than half of 1929 levels. The price of hogs in 1933 was the lowest it had been in more than three decades. The price of cotton in New Orleans, which was already a paltry fourteen cents per pound in 1920, sank to five cents per pound in 1929, with no improvement in the following years; at that price, tenant farmers could not make tenancy or rent payments, or pay down their outstanding debts.[2]

Pervasive industrial unemployment and low agricultural commodity prices left millions of Americans without the means to secure food, clothing, and other basic necessities. The private charities, churches, community chests, and state-run pensions that had formed the country's primary safety net were unable to meet the crushing demand for basic assistance. The Work Bureau, an emergency relief program established by some of New York City's private charities in 1930, paid an average of $15.00 per week to the unemployed; this was a little more than half what an unskilled laborer earned. A similar program in Philadelphia paid $4.00 per day in late 1930, but a year later could manage only $4.39 per week. Bread lines, soup kitchens, and other charitable endeavors sprang up all over the United States, attempting to provide in food what they could not provide in cash.

Mass unemployment, homelessness, hunger, and deprivation led the federal government to assume unprecedented responsibilities in banking, housing, agriculture, industry, health, education, and social welfare; it also brought federal support to school meal programs for the first time. The infusion of federal monies into what had previously been locally, often privately funded initiatives had major implications for both policy and implementation. Over the course of the 1930s, school meal programs remained the primary means of addressing malnutrition among children at the population level, but they also became the foundation of a demand-side solution to the "farm problem," creating considerable tension between health promotion and agricultural protection, and between food security and farm sustainability.

During the 1920s and 1930s, federal administrations regarded with considerable concern the growing gap between the agricultural and industrial economies. Unlike industrial markets, agricultural markets are largely inelastic: the demand for food is unaffected by fluctuations in price. Whether food is cheap or expensive, consumption levels are generally stable relative to the size of the population. Bumper crops were thus a problem in unregulated markets, for increases in supply drove down prices without a concurrent increase in demand; in other words, as farmers produced more food, they risked reducing their profits, a paradox of the agricultural economy in which gains in efficiency were punished with drops in price. In extreme cases, prices deflated so much that the costs of growing, harvesting, and transporting exceeded the market value of the crops. Combined with high fixed costs—the need to invest heavily in land and machinery—and the unpredictability of growing conditions, agriculture was an especially vulnerable part of the nation's economy.

Ironically, the farm problem resulted in part from heavy investment, both public and private, in the development of labor-saving technologies and the scientific study of agriculture and animal husbandry. Farmers in the early twentieth century had better seeds and better methods for controlling diseases and pests than they had in the nineteenth century. The widespread adoption of Mendelian hybridization, especially the production of high-yield hybrid corn, produced hardier, more bountiful crops. The Haber-Bosch process made cheap, synthetic nitrogen fertilizer widely available after World War I and, along with increased mechanization, enhanced the scale and efficiency of commodity farming and monoculture. Although these developments raised the start-up costs of farming, they vastly improved yields, leading to production levels often in excess of what domestic and international markets could support. Between 1917 and 1929, farm output in the United States increased 13 percent with no signs of slowing.[3]

By the time the Depression struck, the larger farms were already overproducing many agricultural commodities, creating surpluses of food at a time when millions were going hungry. Many farmers resorted to destroying excess produce or leaving it to rot in the fields because consumers could not afford to buy it at prices sufficient to cover the costs of harvesting and marketing. The sociologist Janet Poppendieck has argued that "the paradox of want amid plenty" during the Depression became "a central symbol of the irrationality of the economic system."[4]

Although the coexistence of surplus foods with widespread hunger and malnutrition had been a problem prior to the Depression, the conditions of the 1930s made both problems worse. Millions of people were unemployed, and many more were underemployed, leading them to substitute cheaper foods for meat, milk, fresh fruits and vegetables, and other expensive foodstuffs while those very items abounded in fields and storehouses. Consumers could not afford to buy, and producers could not afford to sell. Between 1929 and 1934, industrial production diminished 42 percent but prices decreased only 15 percent; agricultural production dropped only 15 percent but prices fell 40 percent.[5] School meal programs ultimately became a stabilizing mechanism in the agricultural economy by providing a new market for excess foods, but this privileged the economic role of such programs over their role in health and education.

This incorporation of school meals into national agricultural policy had two main phases. In the first phase, the federal government, along with local and state governments, set up emergency relief systems to purchase surplus foods and distribute them to schools, providing economic support for farmers and feeding hungry children. In the second phase, which is discussed in the next chapter, reformers sought legislation to create permanent federal support for school meal programs. These efforts ultimately resulted in the National School Lunch Act, an entitlement passed in 1946 to provide states with federal funding for school meal programs.

The National School Lunch Act ultimately reflected the tensions and ambiguities that surrounded health, education, social welfare, and agriculture in national politics during the Depression and, to a lesser extent, during World War II. The act's twofold goal—"to safeguard the health and well-being of the Nation's children and to encourage the domestic consumption of nutritious agricultural commodities"—firmly hitched the interests of consumers (schoolchildren) to those of producers (farms, ranches, and dairies).[6] This legislation purported to address both the food problem and the farm problem, but the two agendas were not equally represented. Malnutrition and hunger became little more than a justification for what was otherwise an agricultural price-protection measure. Concern about malnourishment had propelled the development of school meal programs, but it was agricultural economics that ultimately secured permanent federal funding for them.

There were several reasons for this shift in priorities. First, prominent fiascos involving surplus crops—such as withholding federal grain stores from drought victims or destroying excess food at taxpayer expense while families starved—along with the rhetoric of hunger in a land of plenty, firmly connected the farm problem and the food problem for the American public and made it politically favorable to legislate the utilization, rather than the destruction, of surpluses. Indeed, schools became the mechanism by which surplus foods, purchased with tax revenue, became a return on investment rather than a casualty of agricultural success.

Second, the lack of a widely accepted metric for measuring hunger or malnutrition in populations called into question the reliability of existing data. Congress, rather than physicians and health authorities, ultimately evaluated the validity of the evidence that a significant proportion of American children were malnourished. Despite overwhelming medical opinion that hunger and malnutrition were common and posed a significant health problem, Congress questioned whether malnutrition was a health problem important enough or extensive enough to require federal intervention.

Lastly, many in Congress fought to oppose federal interference in public health and education, both of which were traditionally within the purview of the states. Despite the sweeping changes ushered in during the New Deal, the specter of socialism continued to haunt many health and welfare initiatives, and school meal programs were no exception. Conventional political tensions—for example, between states' rights and federal expansion or between southern Democrats and northern Republicans—along with congressional agriculture committees focused more on commercial advancement and food security than on human health or dietary needs, produced school lunch legislation heavy on agricultural protection and light on nutritional promotion. Despite the prominent place of hunger and malnutrition among the deprivations wrought by the Depression, the federal government shifted the purpose of school meal programs away from public health nutrition and toward agricultural protection. While this also made school meal programs available to more children than ever before, many who needed them most remained excluded due to the perpetuation of racial and socioeconomic inequalities that remained unaddressed by the National School Lunch Act.

But what brought school meals once again to national attention was less about children's nutritional health—as had been the case during World War I—and more about the role of the federal government in disaster relief. Just as the harsh realities of the Depression began to set in, the nation experienced what Secretary of Agriculture Arthur Hyde deemed "the worst drought ever recorded." Concentrated in the Ohio and Mississippi River Valleys, the drought of 1930 affected more than half of the states in the nation, extending from Texas to Pennsylvania and Virginia to Montana. High temperatures and low rainfall caused forest fires to burn uncontrollably, rivers to dry up, hydroelectric plants to close, and wildlife to perish; by the end of the summer, even wells were running dry. Health authorities reported with alarm an increase in the morbidity and mortality rates of infants and children in states heavily affected by the drought. Agricultural output plummeted, and the average farm income dropped 25 percent. The American Red Cross stated that it had "never been confronted by a disaster of larger proportions" and even suspended its policy of not providing relief for crop disasters.[7]

As winter approached, many rural families worried about the survival of their livestock and the feeding of their children. Urbanites marveled that farmers could be without food, but a reliance on monoculture, especially in the cotton and tobacco fields of the South and the corn and wheat fields of the Great Plains, had largely replaced subsistence farming in much of the country. Between the drought and the Depression, most sharecroppers and tenant farmers did not have the resources to survive the winter, let alone resume farming in the spring. Livestock had to be killed for food when pasturage dried up, and the failure of banks and lending institutions meant that credit was generally unavailable.[8] Although Herbert Hoover did more than any previous president to provide federal assistance during an economic depression, he remained committed to a policy of nonintervention in the economy. Instead of government regulation, bureaucratic expansion, or large federal expenditures, he promoted "collective self-help," state-based relief, and private-sector initiatives such as the Red Cross, cooperative agricultural marketing associations, and natural resource conservation. Though federal relief did finally come in 1931, most regarded it as too little, too late, and Hoover's reputation as the "Great Humanitarian" was considerably tarnished.[9]

Against this backdrop, another congressional debate took place over whether to distribute food from federal holdings to the hungry. Surplus agricultural products that the Federal Farm Board had purchased from growers—a price-protection measure undertaken with the knowledge that the products would eventually have to be "dumped" on foreign markets at a loss or simply dumped—filled federal storehouses. By March of 1931 there were 250 million bushels of wheat in federal possession, enough to bake over 15 billion loaves of bread.[10] Though purchased from farmers with taxpayer money to stabilize the wheat market, the surpluses were not distributed to the taxpaying hungry, initially because the Federal Farm Board did not have the authority to do so.

When the issue came before Congress in late 1930, support and opposition split much the way it did in the drought relief debates. The question of whether to release surplus grain hinged on several issues, including the perceived severity of hunger and malnutrition and the concern that distributing wheat stores would depress prices even further, effectively feeding the hungry at the expense of farmers' incomes. It was not until March of 1932 that Congress finally authorized surplus foods to be released to the American Red Cross, at no charge, for distribution to the unemployed and the destitute. Not only did this not cause a drastic drop in wheat prices, as many politicians had feared—the decline in the price of wheat was comparable to price fluctuations in other commodities—but the surpluses did indeed feed the hungry poor. They were in such high demand, in fact, that within three months many regions were already applying for additional allotments.[11]

This marked the first time that Congress considered a food assistance measure, and though it was ultimately a small one in comparison with those to come, it set the tone for future discussions of food aid. Both the Senate and the House "clearly defined their responsibility as that of protecting the interests of the commercial farmer," Poppendieck argued. "Neither suggested that an agriculture committee might be charged with a broader responsibility for the way that the nation was fed. . . . Despite much nostalgia about farming as a way of life, it had become a business, and the agriculture committees of Congress saw their task as that of ensuring or enhancing the profitability of that business and protecting it in its interaction with other sectors of the economy."[12] When Congress later debated the role of the federal government in school lunch programs—and the degree to which such programs should develop with agricultural interests in mind—many of the same issues remained central.

Although drought relief and food aid were only two of the many reasons that Hoover's once-bright public image dimmed, they were especially memorable ones. When the Depression continued to worsen in spite of—and in the case of higher tariffs because of—Hoover's economic policies, in 1932 Americans elected to office Franklin Roosevelt, the first Democrat to win a popular majority in the presidential election since 1856. Roosevelt rejected laissez-faire governance and embarked on a course of extensive federal regulation and intervention. In 1933, he signed into law legislation that dispensed relief money to the poor, created jobs, protected labor unions, and raised farm prices. Roosevelt's policies made the federal government a key participant in economic regulation, agricultural market control, labor relations, business practice, public works, health care, and social welfare.

Like Hoover, Roosevelt made a public relations blunder in negotiating between agricultural price control and food relief. One of the first pieces of New Deal legislation passed, the Agricultural Adjustment Act established a "domestic allotment" system for farmers. In essence, the federal government paid farmers (with a consumer tax) to decrease production of seven commodities—corn, cotton, dairy, hogs, rice, tobacco, and wheat—and in the case of periodic surpluses, purchased excess crops at protected prices. This shifted federal farm policy from supply control, as practiced by the Federal Farm Board under Hoover, to production control, which ultimately had more success reducing surpluses, controlling prices, and securing the participation of farmers.

In the summer of 1933, just after Roosevelt signed the act into law, it was already too late to pay farmers not to produce. Fearing bumper crops of corn, cotton, and hogs, the Agricultural Adjustment Administration instead paid farmers to plow under 10 million acres of cotton—a quarter of the national total—then bought and slaughtered over 6 million hogs. Once again, the federal government did not dispense surplus commodities to the needy, but instead destroyed them at taxpayer expense, removing them from the market entirely. The reasoning was much the same as it had been two years earlier: many feared that the mass distribution of food would depress the agricultural economy even further, and there existed no agreed-upon estimates of the extent or severity of hunger and malnutrition.

The perceived failure of the federal government to distribute surplus foods to the needy was due less to callous disregard for American suffering than to the complexity of the farm economy. When the Federal Surplus Relief Corporation—established in late 1933 after the public outcry elicited by the Agricultural Adjustment Administration's policies—began to distribute surplus commodities to the states for use in relief efforts, it became clear that doing so was not as simple as brokering the transfer of excess, unsaleable foods from farmers to those unable to afford sufficient sustenance. The FSRC had to balance the demands of various constituents, which included not only farmers and the hungry unemployed but also competing producers, food processors, wholesale and retail grocers, food marketers and transporters, relief administrators at the local, state, and federal levels, and taxpayers.[13]

To make matters worse, no federal agency defined exactly what counted as a "surplus" commodity. Although surplus commodity distribution came to be an ever more significant part of federal food relief, the plowing under of useable cotton and the slaughter of healthy hogs remained a bitter memory for many Americans, evidence that the government's agricultural policies often seemed insane. Indeed, locked storehouses overflowing with grain, fertile fields plowed under, and the mass slaughter of healthy hogs remained potent images long after the episodes themselves occurred. The Almanac Singers, a folk band that included Woody Guthrie and Pete Seeger, referenced the events a decade later in the antiwar song "Plow Under":

Remember when the AAA
Killed a million hogs a day?
Instead of hogs it's men today.
Plow the fourth one under.[14]

In the political context of the debates then occurring about American involvement in the war in Europe and the historical context of federal agricultural policies, to "plow under," a once-innocuous farming practice done to maintain the health of farmland, came to represent a senseless or callous act.

The federal government became increasingly involved in food relief as the Depression worsened, but surpluses were generally distributed to individuals and families rather than to schools or other community institutions. As a result, many cities created emergency funds to feed poor and malnourished children. In 1930, Detroit began to provide free meals to poor schoolchildren, and schools reduced the price of a half-pint bottle of milk from five cents to three cents.[15] St. Louis established an Emergency Lunch Room Fund of $25,000 in 1931 "for the purpose of furnishing lunches at less than cost to such public school pupils of compulsory school age as would otherwise be unable, by reason of insufficient nutrition, to attend school and pursue the courses of study prescribed."[16] By 1932, numerous cities across the country bolstered their existing meal programs—or elected to start them for the first time—to address issues of hunger and malnutrition. Indeed, there was convincing evidence that malnourishment was increasing. A longitudinal study conducted in Pittsburgh, for example, found that the proportion of schoolchildren who were significantly underweight began increasing in 1928. Between 1923 and 1927, the percentage of children 14 percent or more below the average weight was consistently around 7 percent; by 1932, it had risen incrementally to 12.6 percent.[17]

Cities also relied on the generosity of their citizens to help those in need. Beginning in 1930, Superintendent of Schools William O'Shea asked New York City teachers to donate 5 percent of their salaries—and any time they could spare—to the "war against hunger and starvation." Between 1930 and 1934, when state relief funds became available, more than $4 million was contributed to the School Relief Fund. Along with WPA labor, which helped supply tables and benches for students to use, and donations from the gas companies of laundry stoves, which were the only available stoves suitable for large-scale cooking, the city was able to supply free meals daily to over 45,000 children at eighty schools. All of the money contributed by teachers went to providing as much food as possible to schoolchildren.[18] "There was none of the care-free spirit of a picnic," a reporter for the *New York Times* observed at one of the schools, "but gray walls and sober-minded children eating to live."[19] The generosity of New York City's teachers kept thousands of children from starving during one of the worst winters on record: the temperatures were so cold that the Niagara Falls froze solid, something that typically occurs only once every few decades.

Rural schools continued much as they had previously. The agricultural economy had been badly depressed since the end of World War I, and rural schools were already accustomed to working with limited resources. Nevertheless, the Depression made things even worse, and many schools were unable to maintain their meal programs. In Wisconsin, for example, nearly half of the rural and state graded schools served food in 1924, but only a third still did so in 1933.[20] During the early 1930s, rural schools, as they had during the previous decade, sought ways to develop or maintain meal services with low or nonexistent funds, makeshift equipment, and whatever food was available. At consolidated schools, which had larger student bodies and better resources than one-room schools, cooperative cafeterias became a common response to financial difficulties.

At the Cherry Valley Central School in New York, many children left home at 8 A.M. on school days and did not return until 5 P.M. due to the long distances traveled to and from school. Combined with the deepening need created by extremely low farm prices, the school began a cooperative cafeteria in December of 1932 with the aim of serving one hot dish each day to supplement the foods brought from home. Each dish sold for two cents, but the school also set up a program in which children could donate raw produce from their farms and gardens and receive cooked food in exchange. The school sent weekly newsletters to parents, detailing the menus for the following week and establishing the "exchange value" of different farm products; the school essentially set up its own agricultural market, not unlike today's Farm-to-School program. According to school authorities, the families participating in the exchange program "received a better price for their produce than the retailer could give them." Of the 160 children at the school, 60 paid for their meals with food credits, 70 paid cash, and 15 received free meals from the Parent-Teacher Association; only 15 children elected not to participate.[21]

But not all health and education authorities supported the establishment of school meal programs. Ada Newman, a public health nurse
in Wisconsin, argued in 1932 against the distribution of food (except-
ing milk) in schools even if privately financed. "By feeding children in
school," she cautioned, "we open the way for the Poor Commissioner
to cut still further on the diet sent into the home."[22] Newman's concern about the effects on relief distribution if it were diluted across
various agencies and points of contact was not an uncommon one.
The shortcomings of the school as a site for intervention were widely
recognized, and some health authorities worried that intervening in
an institution that most children attended fewer than half the days in
a year would create the appearance of food and nutrition security but
would actually undercut it.

Despite these concerns, federal agencies increasingly developed
relief distribution models that incorporated key institutions. The
Federal Emergency Relief Association, for example, oversaw the distribution of grants to the states for use in relief programs such as unemployment compensation, food and clothing distribution, and health
services. In 1933, the association authorized states to distribute federal
monies to schools for the hiring of unemployed women to prepare and
serve food in schools. "With probably 6,000,000 children in the homes
of the unemployed now on our relief lists and with the difficulty of
providing adequate and proper food for children in the homes," wrote
Harry Hopkins, director of the Federal Emergency Relief Association, "I am anxious that safeguards be established to the fullest extent
against malnutrition among children."[23] In Knox County, Tennessee,
where 11,000 rural children attended eighty-three schools, association funds helped expand the number of school lunch programs from
sixteen to seventy.[24] By 1935, the association was subsidizing labor
costs for school lunch programs in thirty-nine states, employing 7,400
women to feed 1.9 million schoolchildren per week.[25]

In 1935, the newly formed Works Progress Administration (WPA)[26]
assumed this duty from the Federal Emergency Relief Association.
The WPA was a work relief agency that put the unemployed to work
on public projects. WPA workers built roads, hospitals, and schools,
created and maintained parks, installed public art projects, provided

child care, and performed numerous other tasks in industry, agriculture, government, and the arts; the WPA also trained—through local colleges and extension services—and employed thousands of women to prepare and serve lunches to schoolchildren, one of the agency's "most popular programs."[27]

Even with WPA involvement, local authorities retained most of the responsibility for operating school lunch programs. Space, power, water, equipment, and food all had to be provided by the school board, PTA, or other sponsoring organization—as in the previous decades. The WPA paid the salaries of all cooks and servers at participating schools, accounting for approximately one-quarter to one-third of the total operating expenses of a school meal program. Within a year, thirty-six states, the District of Columbia, and New York City were receiving federal employment support for their lunch programs. In Mississippi, for example, an exceptionally poor and mostly rural state that had very few school lunch programs prior to 1936, the WPA provided assistance in all eighty-three counties; with the help of roughly two thousand women employed by the agency, more than a thousand schools subsequently provided lunches for 75,000 children.[28]

While the WPA provided labor assistance to schools operating lunch programs, amendments to the Agricultural Adjustment Act passed in August of 1935 provided a legislative basis for the distribution of surplus foods to schools free of charge. Under Section 32, the act authorized the secretary of agriculture to appropriate 30 percent of customs receipts to "encourage the domestic consumption of [agricultural] commodities or products by diverting them, by the payment of benefits or indemnities or by other means, from the normal channels of trade and commerce or by increasing their utilization through benefits, indemnities, donations or by other means."[29] This empowered the USDA to divert price-depressing commodities (usually surpluses) from agricultural markets by purchasing them directly and disposing of them either in foreign countries or in domestic relief programs (see figure 3). The Agricultural Adjustment Act did not, however, establish a mechanism for the purpose of achieving this redistribution of surplus foods to achieve price control; nor did it include standards for measuring the performance of such duties.

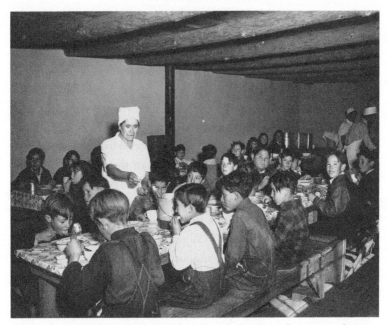

Figure 3. A WPA worker serves lunch made from surplus commodities to schoolchildren in Penasco, New Mexico.

Source: Irving Rusinow, "Taos County, New Mexico. The hot lunch, school at Penasco," 1941, National Archives, Record Group 83, "Records of the Bureau of Agricultural Economics, 1876–1959," NAI 521840.

Shortly after these amendments became law, the Federal Surplus Relief Corporation, the independent federal agency that had previously overseen the distribution of surpluses, was incorporated into the USDA and renamed the Federal Surplus Commodities Corporation. This consolidation and name change represented the beginning of a merger between price-protection measures for commercial agriculture and food relief, with the latter becoming a mechanism for—and thus dependent upon—the former. In its first annual report, the new agency declared "that the Corporation's greatest value was not as a relief organization, but rather as an agency to assist the Department of Agriculture in the execution of surplus removal programs."[30]

Initially, the USDA diverted excess foods to state relief agencies for distribution directly to poor individuals and families who were on the relief registers, but in 1939, schools became for the first time a regular recipient of agricultural surpluses. This shift "would not only provide health-building lunches for millions of needy children," wrote Milo Perkins, the president of the Federal Surplus Commodities Corporation and associate administrator of the USDA's Surplus Marketing Administration (SMA), "but would also provide additional outlets for agricultural commodities."[31] This policy change resulted in a significant escalation of federal involvement in school meal programs, as the SMA diverted agricultural products that were previously sold overseas to domestic schools instead. With tensions mounting in Europe, many foreign markets could no longer absorb American surpluses to the same extent they had previously, and the USDA found in schools a new domestic outlet for unsaleable produce.[32]

The SMA, which oversaw the distribution of surplus foods to schools, appointed personnel to the states to facilitate communication between federal authorities and state boards of education, local school districts, PTAs, and other groups involved in school meal programs. To receive surplus foods, the agency operating the local program was required to consent to certain terms. First, sponsors agreed not to curtail their usual food purchases. The surplus foods were to supplement, not replace, locally available foods, allowing schools to expand the number of meals served, increase variety, and keep costs down. Second, sponsors could not charge "certified" children for the lunches they ate. Certified children were those whom local school or health authorities identified as in need of supplemental feeding due to financial hardship or poor health. Third, schools could not distinguish between paying and nonpaying children, either in the manner of service or in the meals served. Most schools adopted a system of tickets or tokens, which paying children could purchase and certified children could receive free of charge, so that no money changed hands in the lunchroom itself. While it is unlikely that this method fooled any children, who must have known which of their peers were on the relief registers, it at least kept up the pretense of socioeconomic equality and may have curtailed the potential for stigmatization. Lastly, sponsors could not operate lunchrooms for profit; any receipts in excess of costs had to be reinvested in the lunch program itself. As long as these conditions were met, any school or school district could receive free foods simply by applying directly to the SMA.[33]

Areas with badly depressed economies and few existing meal programs were the primary beneficiaries of this initiative. In March of 1940, only 19 percent of the schools participating had initiated meal programs before SMA assistance became available, and nearly 40 percent of the participating children were from families receiving local, state, or federal relief.[34] Though primarily a price-control measure designed to bolster agricultural incomes, the SMA school lunch program embraced the health of children as a commensurate goal. It addressed "a very real need in the communities," Perkins noted, "while providing an unusually good outlet for commodities in which expanded domestic markets are essential for farmers."[35]

This raised two questions about the SMA program: Did it increase the income of farmers, and did it improve the health of children? Both questions were (and remain) difficult to answer conclusively due to the lack of sufficient data and the complexity of factors involved. Using records gathered from a sample of schools during March of 1941—March typically saw the highest level of participation—the SMA estimated that the distribution of surplus foods to school lunch programs increased farmers' gross incomes by at least $2 million. This was a small amount relative to the $9 billion in total income generated by farms in 1940, but the actual increase was likely much higher. The SMA's figure accounts only for the food bought and distributed to schools, not for the higher prices created or maintained by government purchasing programs, nor for the expansion of markets generated by food redistribution.[36] Geoffrey Shepherd, professor of economics at Iowa State College, estimated the real gain in farmers' incomes resulting from the SMA school lunch program to be considerably more than the USDA spent on surplus removal. He calculated that in the fiscal year ending 30 June 1941, when the federal government spent $14.8 million to purchase 341 million pounds of food, farm incomes increased between $16 and $29 million.[37]

Improvements in nutritional health were also difficult to assess, but there was clear evidence of the need for improvement. In Missouri, for example, physicians employed by the Civil Works Administration inspected almost 300,000 school children in 1934 and considered 14 percent of them malnourished.[38] Dietary surveys, which evaluated nutritional health from the supply side, also became increasingly common. According to data collected by the U.S. Departments of Agriculture and Labor in 1936–1937, more than a third of the families surveyed— "representative nonrelief families, each with a husband and wife, both native-born"—had diets that did not meet the minimum standards established by nutritionists.[39] Studies of impoverished and disenfranchised groups revealed considerably higher rates of malnourishment and dietary insufficiency.[40] Perhaps most damning, military rejection statistics during World War II were even higher than those during World War I, and malnutrition remained a significant cause of inadequacy.[41]

Anecdotal evidence and small-scale studies continued to show that children who received school lunches on a regular basis were healthier and performed better in school than those who did not. In the state of Washington, "educators, classroom teachers, social workers, and all engaged in child welfare activities agree that better work habits and attitudes, as well as better attendance, result from regular school lunches."[42] A study conducted by the South Carolina Agricultural Experiment Station found that children who ate a complete school lunch had better growth and development than those who received only supplemental foods at school.[43] Lucille Watson, the Georgia state director of school lunch programs, received letters extolling the benefits of school lunches. "They have had 50 percent less sickness in our school and we have had 40 to 50 percent better attendance," wrote one teacher from a small mill village. "Their general attitude is 75 percent better."[44]

The SMA school lunch program expanded in response to demand, which was overwhelming. Between 1939, when the program began, and 1941, the number of schools participating increased threefold, the number of children served increased fivefold, and the amount of food distributed increased tenfold. In March of 1942, when the program peaked, the SMA was supplying surplus commodities to 93,000 schools serving 6 million children. More than 40 percent of the nation's schools and nearly a quarter of school-aged children received surplus foods in their school lunches.[45]

Although the SMA school lunch program improved farm incomes and likely improved the health of many children, there were several drawbacks, and experiences at the local level temper the conclusions drawn from national data. Distribution of surplus commodities, for instance, differed widely across the states. The percentage of schoolchildren served ranged from 61.7 percent in Georgia to 1.5 percent in Rhode Island. In general, the program was most heavily utilized in states with badly depressed agricultural economies, especially in the South and West, where cash crop monoculture had largely replaced more diversified farming practices.[46]

Because the SMA program was an outgrowth of agricultural policy rather than public health, it did not include nutritional standards or guidelines. This was left completely to local discretion. A survey of lunch programs in the District of Columbia and select counties of Illinois, Kansas, Massachusetts, Pennsylvania, and Wisconsin revealed tremendous variation in the composition of school meals. The lunches in Iron County, Wisconsin, for example, averaged just 310 calories, while those in Neosho County, Kansas, were nearly four times larger at 1,180 calories. Milk consumption varied even more, from 0.2 quarts per child per month in Williamson County, Illinois, to 5.5 quarts per child per month in Washington, DC. This was due in part to seasonal variation—participation tended to be high in the winter months and lower in the fall and spring—and in part to changes in available surpluses and uneven distribution.[47]

The kinds of foods available also fluctuated radically from year to year. For example, drought in the Midwest caused beef to be in surplus during 1935 and 1936, accounting for 59 percent and 31 percent, respectively, of surplus foods distributed to state relief agencies in those years. In each of the three years following, meat comprised less than 1 percent of the food disbursed. Dairy products made up only 10 percent of the available surplus in 1936, but 39 percent in 1938.[48] Similar trends continued even as schools became the primary recipients for surplus produce. This made dietetic skill even more important; schools with lunch supervisors trained in nutrition could more easily adapt to significant fluctuations in available foods. Similarly, schools or districts with more robust local markets could better offset imbalances in surplus produce with local purchases.

In addition, while the policy of the SMA was to distribute available foods only upon request, many participants complained that schools became a dumping ground for unsaleable surpluses. In Virginia, for example, the SMA sent "loads of onions or grapefruit or what not to various communities." State Superintendent of Education Sidney Hall argued that "the people there did not need those commodities. We needed a person who knew nutritional values, who would select foods according to the welfare and the needs of the children, and then if, perchance, the Surplus Commodities Corporation had some surplus food that fitted into that program of nutrition, they then should have been ordered."[49] The SMA provided foods but no specific guidance on how to employ them effectively, and those foods often required substantial preparation or combination with other foods to make them palatable. Few children want to eat a raw onion, and a delivery of onions and grapefruit does not provide a very good basis for a meal, even in the hands of a trained dietitian.

Although states continued to utilize extension services and university departments of home economics to publish literature, give lectures and demonstrations, and train workers, most schools did not have regular access to a nutritionist or dietitian. Indeed, the majority of state health departments did not employ such a person. It wasn't until the 1950s that most states did, and only three—Massachusetts, New York, and Connecticut—could claim uninterrupted employment of at least one nutritionist between 1930 and 1950.[50] Many state boards of education expressed a need for more training in how to operate a school lunch program, citing a shortage of local expertise. Of the roughly 221,000 schools in the country, only about 18,000 had a home economics teacher.[51] In most cases, only the largest school districts could afford to hire personnel whose sole responsibility was management of the meal program.

This made commodity dumping especially problematic, as without the benefit of skilled preparation and combination, many children grew tired of eating the same foods over and over again. George

Chatfield, then a member of the New York City Board of Education, recalled "when [the USDA] said we have got to have apples. Do you know where they went? They came so frequently in the lunch program that they went in the toilets. The kids didn't eat them."[52] According to the chair of the Community School-Lunch Project of the National Congress of Parents and Teachers, one school district in South Carolina "had nothing but eggs for a whole month, shipped down to South Carolina from Maine, and when our South Carolina hens are laying just as many eggs as Maine hens are laying."[53] The supervisor of school cafeterias in Rockville, Maryland, pointed out that surplus foods were only useful if the children recognized them as foods. One of her districts received six crates of surplus grapefruit, "but the children of that district come from homes which have never used grapefruit and hence haven't cultivated a taste for it. So the children use the grapefruit to play catch with."[54] One could argue, as some members of Congress did, that this indicated an overestimation of actual hunger or starvation—surely children who were truly hungry would eat whatever they could get—but much of the malnourishment identified by health authorities was traced less to lack of total food than to diets that were not sufficiently varied or that consistently lacked certain kinds of food.[55]

The availability of storage facilities also limited the extent to which schools could receive surplus foods. Perishable foods, such as milk and fresh fruits and vegetables, typically required refrigerated storage areas unless they could be utilized immediately. Even less perishable commodities took up space, a premium in many cities. The United Neighborhood Houses of New York City, which served lunches to poor children, had to turn down a shipment of surplus potatoes because they had nowhere to put them. "We had to take what was available," said a representative of the organization, "and use it to the best ability we could."[56] While they did not mind the variability of supply, they were constrained by the need to store foods prior to use.

One solution to the problem of transporting and storing fresh produce was to can excess perishable foods. "Few of the [school] cafeterias are equipped to store and prepare the [surplus] food," observed a nutritionist from California. "Many items could be used to better advantage if they were processed before delivery, thereby eliminating additional labor and expensive equipment."[57] In the mid-1930s, the WPA began canning and drying surplus foods for use in school lunch programs and other food relief initiatives. On average, the WPA canned over 10 million quarts and dried over 2 million pounds of food every year.[58]

School gardens were another solution to the same problem, as they eliminated the need for long-range transportation. This became particularly important with the rationing of gasoline during World War II. The WPA, along with some state relief agencies, hired workers to plant and maintain community and school gardens and to can produce to increase the variety and quantity of foods incorporated in school lunch programs. In the summer of 1942, for example, 530 acres of school gardens in Minnesota, combined with donations, made available to the schools 350,000 quarts of canned vegetables, 3,000 quarts of canned fruit, 19 tons of dried food, 440 tons of stored food, and 1,500 pounds of frozen food.[59] Los Angeles County had 1,000 acres of community gardens under cultivation; with one worker per acre, the fields could produce at harvest time more than 3 million pounds of vegetables monthly and 600 cases of canned goods daily.[60]

School gardening dates at least to the late nineteenth century, but it was seldom a part of school lunch programs prior to the 1940s. Kansas City, for example, had over sixty school gardens in 1914, and many of those schools also had lunch programs. Children worked in the gardens voluntarily, as an extracurricular activity, then chose either to bring the produce home or to donate it to charities or hospitals; none was used in the lunch programs.[61] In rural areas, school gardens were typically used to teach agricultural techniques and practices. In neither urban nor rural schools were gardens a significant source of food for school lunch programs until the 1930s, in part because of the labor needed to grow large amounts of produce. Gardens require the most tending during the spring and summer months, when schools were not in session. Moreover, harvesting and preserving enough food for even part of the school lunch program was both laborious and time-consuming; children could not do these tasks exclusively during school hours, for it would detract from their studies.

This change in the use of school gardens was due largely to the decrease in surplus foods that resulted from World War II. Agricultural products that had once cost more to harvest than they were worth found lucrative markets in the military and in federally funded foreign aid programs. According to a pamphlet issued by the U.S. Office of Education, "Food supplies raised in school gardens will release comparable amounts of commercially grown crops for our armed forces and our industrial centers, and for the people of allied countries, and will also lessen transportation and distribution problems."[62] Even before the United States entered the war, roughly 17 percent of the schools receiving surplus commodities from the SMA also had gardens or canning projects associated with the lunch program.[63] By 1943, the agricultural surplus that had become the primary source of food for most school meal programs no longer existed, making "victory gardens" not only an important part of the war effort but also a crucial source of food for schoolchildren.[64] In Lake Stevens, Washington, for example,

> [the] policy has been to furnish a well-balanced and nutritious lunch at a low cost. The children in our community come from homes of working people or laboring class, for the most part, and in the past their incomes have been low. Our lunch program has helped a great deal. For the past 4 years we have had school gardens and have frozen perishable vegetables as well as small fruits. This year we have 3,300 pounds of fruits and vegetables frozen. It practically all came from our gardens or from the immediate community.[65]

According to one estimate, victory gardens produced 40 percent of the vegetables Americans consumed in 1945.[66]

With the agricultural surplus gone to the war effort and the rationing of food and fuel, many schools faced the possibility that their lunch programs would have to be curtailed or discontinued completely. Fully a quarter of the schools receiving donated commodities from the SMA relied exclusively on the donations to supply their lunch programs.[67] In most cases, this was due to a lack of cooking apparatus, and so schools served donated fruits and vegetables raw, along with milk, to supplement the lunches children brought from home.

Despite the many challenges that schools faced in utilizing surplus commodities—and many educators and health experts were critical of the system's shortcomings—federal school meal programs were wildly popular. The prospect that support for school meals might end led to a concerted push for legislation that would support such programs in perpetuity. Yet as the next chapter explores, providing permanent federal support for school meal programs proved far more difficult than providing temporary relief during an economic crisis. What was once a humble initiative to improve children's nutrition and increase academic performance became the center of a protracted and contentious debate over the extent of hunger and malnourishment, civil rights, and the proper role of the federal government in education, health, and social welfare.

Chapter 6

From Aid to Entitlement

Creation of the National School Lunch Program

With American entry into World War II, the last vestiges of the Great Depression were effectively quashed. Unemployment fell to less than 10 percent, agricultural surpluses became a boon rather than a liability, and industrial production accelerated. Yet most recognized that wartime spending lifted the country out of the Depression only by running up the national debt, effectively trading one economic problem for another. After the cancellation of many New Deal programs, most notably the WPA, parents and schools became increasingly concerned about the future viability of their school meal programs in the absence of subsidized food and labor.

To prevent schools from closing their lunchrooms, Congress authorized the USDA to switch from a commodity distribution program to a cash indemnity system at the beginning of the 1942–1943 school year. Instead of giving food purchased with Section 32 funds directly to the schools, the USDA instead reimbursed a certain proportion of purchased foods, up to $50 million per year nationwide. Participating schools bought food locally, then submitted a claim to the USDA. The rate of reimbursement depended upon the type of lunch served, with minimum standards set by the USDA's Nutrition Division. Schools could receive nine cents for each Type A Lunch—a half pint of milk, two ounces of protein, one cup of vegetables or fruit, one slice of whole-grain or enriched bread, and two teaspoons of butter or margarine fortified with vitamin A—and six cents for each Type B Lunch, which had the same amount of milk as a Type A Lunch but half of everything else. (The Type B lunch was a complete meal for young children or a supplement for older children.) The USDA estimated that these reimbursements would cover 60 percent of the cost of food used in the lunches and 50 percent of the total cost.[1]

This was the first time the federal government earmarked money specifically for school meal programs and the first time the USDA imposed a nutritional threshold for participation, although many local school boards had long since established minimum nutrition standards to ensure that children did not choose unbalanced or unhealthful meals for themselves. The Type A concept originated from the practice of teachers in an Akron, Ohio, school who graded students' lunch trays. As each student exited the food line, the teacher observed the tray and awarded the student an A grade if the meal was complete; if it was missing something, the student received a card whose color indicated what was lacking (e.g., one color indicated milk, another vegetables, and so forth). If a student did not receive an A grade, he or she returned to the lunch counter with the colored card to be exchanged for the corresponding item. This was not just a practice for ensuring the nutritional quality of children's lunches but also an educational exercise, one that enculturated children into a particular system for creating a balanced meal.[2]

The transition from food distribution to cash indemnity had several consequences for participating schools. Although the latter system ensured that the meals served met minimum nutrition standards, far fewer schools were able to participate. At its peak in March of 1942, the SMA supplied food to more than 93,000 schools serving lunches to 6 million children. For the entire year between July of 1944 and June of 1945, fewer than 30,000 schools serving 3.8 million children participated in the cash indemnity program. Although those numbers increased each year, it took until 1947—the year the NSLP began—before 6 million children again received federally subsidized meals.

The steep drop in participation was due to several factors. Because a quarter of the schools participating in the SMA program had no other source of food and typically no kitchen facilities, those schools were incapable of participating in a cash-based system unless local authorities equipped them and took responsibility for organizing and managing a full lunch service. Even for schools that had equipment, the cash indemnity program created hardships. All food had to be purchased in advance, requiring a considerable operating budget. Since reimbursements were rated monthly, schools had to operate lunch programs for as many as twenty-three school days without federal assistance before even applying, and then they had to continue operations with local funds until the rebate arrived. Furthermore, schools could only receive reimbursements if they served complete meals. With the exception of milk, which the USDA sold to schools independently at a discounted price (usually four to six cents per quart), there were no reimbursements or subsidies for supplemental foods.

The cash indemnity system also failed to remove the discrepancies between different states and territories. The USDA subsidized 45.7 percent of school lunches in Hawaii, for example, but only 1.8 percent in Alaska, even though Hawaii had much greater agricultural output per capita. Other gaps between states with similar circumstances, though not quite so large, were notable nonetheless. The USDA funded 33 percent of the lunches in Arizona but only 10.5 percent of those in New Mexico, and 29.7 percent of the meals in Utah but only 13.7 percent of those in Wyoming. Despite the enormous income gap between New York, one of the richest states, and Mississippi, one of the poorest, the USDA funded 18.5 percent of the lunches in the former and 14.8 percent of those in the latter.[3] The many limitations of the cash indemnity system made it considerably more difficult for schools—especially rural schools and poor urban schools—to participate in the federal program.

To make matters worse, WPA labor was no longer available after June of 1943. By 1941, WPA-supported school lunch programs were operating in all forty-eight states, the District of Columbia, and Puerto Rico; 23,000 schools served an average of 2 million lunches per day with the help of 64,000 WPA workers.[4] Two years later, four times as many schools were serving three times as many lunches per day, and school lunch workers accounted for nearly 20 percent of the agency's employees.[5] Between military service and defense work, however, unemployment dropped dramatically in the early 1940s, and Roosevelt disbanded the WPA with an "honorable discharge." Although the WPA and USDA school lunch programs had operated independently—the former supplied only labor, and the latter supplied only food (or later cash), with schools able to participate in either or both—the majority of schools relied on contributions from both agencies to maintain their lunch services.

The cash reimbursements were not meant to be a permanent school lunch program but rather a temporary, wartime extension of the SMA relief system in the absence of large and predictable surpluses. But the impending cessation of federal aid generated considerable public apprehension. "I think it is safe to say," stated Senator George Aiken of Vermont, "that we [in Congress] get more mail . . . on the school-lunch program than on any other subject, including the international situation."[6] The federal school meal programs that emerged from the New Deal enjoyed immense public support, enough that several senators authored bills to establish them as a regular service, not just a temporary relief measure.

Two bills were introduced on the Senate floor in March of 1944, and the Committee on Agriculture and Forestry held hearings to discuss them. The Smith-Ellender Bill (S. 1824), authored by Senators Ellison Smith of South Carolina and Allen Ellender of Louisiana, and the Russell Bill (S. 1820), authored by Senator Richard Russell of Georgia, each sought to secure permanent federal funding for a nationwide school lunch program.

Ellender and Russell, both of whom remained prominent figures in the push for permanent, federal school lunch legislation, had much in common. Conservative southern Democrats, the two senators generally supported New Deal programs that benefited farmers and the poor, electrified rural regions, and brought federal monies to the states, but they remained vehemently opposed to legislation that would infringe on states' rights or eliminate racial segregation. In 1938, both men opposed a federal antilynching bill, which put them in the minority even in the South, and Ellender authored a bill to outlaw interracial marriage, which failed to pass. Despite their general conservatism and overt racism, Russell and Ellender felt deep sympathy for the plight of farmers and evinced genuine concern for the nutritional health of children, leading them to aggressively pursue federal investment in school meal programs.[7] Georgia, South Carolina, and Louisiana also had the first-, second-, and fourth-highest levels of participation in the SMA school lunch initiative, giving those states considerable incentive to secure a continuation of federal involvement.

In general, the two bills were quite similar; each authorized the federal government to grant money and surplus foods to the states for the preparation and serving of meals in schools. The bills differed, though, over financing—the Smith-Ellender bill required matching funds from the states, whereas the Russell bill did not—and over which federal department should have final authority for running the initiative. The Russell Bill, in keeping with tradition, gave managerial authority over the program to the secretary of agriculture; Russell even used the same language as section 32 of the Agricultural Adjustment Act. The Smith-Ellender Bill, in contrast, stated that the secretary of education should oversee the school lunch program and permitted money to be spent on nutrition education as well as feeding.

Education organizations, such as the National Education Association and the National Congress of Parents and Teachers, favored the Smith-Ellender Bill. "If children are to learn proper habits of nutrition which will insure well-nourished bodies as they grow into adulthood," Assistant Commissioner of Education Bess Goodykoontz testified before the Senate Committee on Agriculture and Forestry, "teaching must go along with feeding."[8] Clyde Erwin, the North Carolina state superintendent of education, argued that his state could expand school involvement better under the Office of Education: "We have 1,100 lunchrooms in our State, and we are feeding approximately 250,000 children a day, which is between one-third and one-fourth of the children enrolled in our schools. But out of the 1,100 lunchrooms, only 600 of them are participating in this Federal program."[9]

Nutritionists preferred the Smith-Ellender Bill as well, and it received endorsements from the American Dietetic Association and the American Home Economics Association. According to the latter, "The buying of the food in terms of nutritional values for the children

[was] more carefully supervised [in the Smith-Ellender Bill]," and there seemed to be fewer conflicts of interest between addressing the nutrition needs of school children and protecting farm prices.[10] "If we are to dispose of these surpluses for the benefit of the school children," Ellender himself noted, "it is bound to come into conflict with the plans of diet recommendations." He went on to argue that "the chief object of the Department of Agriculture would be to get rid of such commodities. Now, I can well see where, if we left it to the Department, it might send to certain schools certain commodities that would throw . . . nutrition recommendations all out of balance."[11]

Most other individuals and organizational representatives who testified before the Senate Committee, if they expressed a preference at all, favored the Russell Bill, in large part because it did not require matching funds from the states and was similar to the ongoing temporary programs operated by the USDA. Though criticism of the USDA, especially over indiscriminate commodity dumping, was not uncommon, it was mostly constructive; satisfaction with existing measures was quite high, and many schools were happy to get any federal assistance they could.[12]

What is perhaps most notable about the hearings held before the Senate Committee is that not one person who testified opposed permanent federal legislation. Health, nutrition, and education authorities, community and youth organizations, labor groups, and religious leaders all agreed that the school lunch program should be continued and expanded with financial support from the federal government. "Speaking as a doctor and a public-health officer," Surgeon General Parran stated, "I think there is probably no experiment the Federal Government could make which would have a greater, more beneficial influence on the future health of this country than the appropriations such as are contemplated under the present bill before this Committee."[13]

Outside of Washington, public demand for federal support also remained strong. The journalist Dorothy Thompson, named by *Time* one of the two most influential women in America (the other being Eleanor Roosevelt), gave a moving plea for the continuance of the federal school lunch initiative. "Do you know," she asked the more than 5 million people who listened to her radio program, "that at Army costs every single one of our 30,000,000 school children could be given breakfast and lunch, balanced and nourishing, every school day, at a cost for actual food that would be less than half of what this Nation spent last year for alcoholic beverages?"[14] In addition, nearly every major medical, public health, farm, labor, and education organization in the country officially endorsed a permanent, federally funded school lunch program.[15] "During my service in Congress," observed Virginia representative John Flannagan, chair of the House Committee on Agriculture, "I have never seen a piece of legislation come before the Congress for consideration that had the backing that this bill has from the people from one end of this country to the other."[16]

In both houses of Congress, however, there were lengthy debates about whether the federal government should become permanently involved in financing and managing school lunch programs. Three fundamental questions underlay congressional debates: 1) Were there enough hungry and malnourished schoolchildren in the country to justify federal intervention as a public health measure? 2) Was the program a necessary (or at least significant) component of agricultural price control? 3) Even if the answer to both questions was yes, did the responsibility for school lunch programs lie with the federal government?[17] The first two questions were much the same as those asked just a few years earlier about the efficacy of the SMA school lunch initiative, but where once lawmakers wondered whether school lunches addressed the two problems adequately, they now wondered whether the two problems even existed any longer.

W. H. Sebrell, medical director of the U.S. Public Health Service and a prominent nutritionist, testified before the House Committee on Agriculture that malnutrition remained a pervasive problem. Surgeon General Parran continued to support this claim, and Major General Lewis Hershey, director of the Selective Service, argued that malnutrition was a common cause of unfitness for military service. According to Hershey, 57 percent of military applicants rejected for medical reasons experienced health problems with "some relation to malnutrition."[18]

Because hunger and malnutrition had neither visible symptoms nor a standard diagnostic definition, and there were no accepted tools for mass surveillance, it was virtually impossible for health authorities to indicate quantitatively how important the problem was or to what extent a national school lunch program would improve children's health. "I wish somebody would point out to me one single outstanding physiologist in this or any other country," the physician and Ohio representative Frederick Smith said, "who would declare that the feeding of these school lunches will cure those conditions [resulting from malnutrition] or prevent them or even mitigate them in the slightest degree." Without clear evidence, it was up to Congress to validate malnutrition as a legitimate health concern and school meals as an effective nutrition initiative. Smith himself remained skeptical even of the existence of widespread malnourishment: "The Surgeon General has testified, I understand, regarding the rejections that were made of our inductees [during World War II] because of diseased conditions resulting from malnutrition. The Surgeon General knows, if he is really a practicing physician, which he is not, that there is no truth or foundation whatsoever for that sort of statement."[19]

The question of whether school lunches were a necessary component of farm price-support measures was more one of prediction than of characterization. Although both employment and wages were high and the war had created a vast demand for nearly all agricultural products, eliminating most surpluses, economists did not know what would happen to wages, employment, and prices after the end of the war. "None of us know," Kansas representative Clifford Hope told the House, "what the conditions will be a year from now."[20] This, too, became an issue for Congress to decide.

Most politicians were convinced by expert testimony and personal experience that malnutrition was a pervasive problem and that schools were an excellent domestic market for agricultural produce. Politicians who had direct experience with school lunches in their states almost unanimously favored permanent federal legislation. "I do not know of a single outstanding American in public life who . . . has had an opportunity to observe the [school lunch] program," Flannagan told the House of Representatives, "that has not publicly declared that the continuance of the program is vital to the future welfare of our Republic."[21] Numerous members of Congress saw just as much need for school meals in the future as they had in the past. Some read letters from constituents on the floors of the House and Senate and praised the virtues of a program that led to better health and education for children and better prices for farmers.[22]

Indeed, no members of Congress opposed school meal programs per se, but many, particularly conservative Republicans in the Northeast and Midwest, contested *federal* investment or involvement in the establishment and maintenance of those programs. The congressional debates were not about the desirability of school meals in principle but rather revolved around issues of civil rights, fiscal responsibility, states' rights, and the role of the federal government in education, health, and social welfare.

As early as 1943, Russell pressed for federal legislation that would delineate "the responsibilit[ies] of the federal government, the States, and local school districts for [school lunch programs]."[23] Illinois representative Ralph Church asked the same question of the House: "Is the matter of school lunches an obligation of local communities and of State governments, or is it a Federal obligation?"[24] Many states felt that without federal assistance they would be unable to maintain, or even begin, school lunch programs sufficient to address hunger and malnutrition, which was still pervasive despite the economic improvements of the war years. The state legislature of South Carolina, for example, wrote to "respectfully commend to our Congressmen and Senators the school-lunch program as operated in the State," arguing that the cessation of federal support would "very seriously handicap the school-lunch program now in operation."[25] The question of federal responsibility subsequently evolved along several lines.

Conservative Republicans took a position based upon "tradition." With the war came record-high employment and wages as well as a seemingly boundless market for agricultural products, leading many to argue that the responsibility for feeding children should shift back to parents and local officials. "The local, school authorities everywhere are better able to pay the expenses and the cost of running these school lunches and the parents of the children are better able to buy them than they have ever been," argued New York representative John Taber. "Under all these circumstances we should leave this to the local authorities to run and not have this involved situation of handing the schools a surplus agriculture product when there are no surpluses and pretending to the people that we are promoting welfare of children when we are not."[26] Illinois representative Noah Mason, a career teacher and school administrator, laid out a chain of responsibility according to proximity.

> I understand the American principle is this—that the parents of the children are responsible, in the first place, for the proper feeding of their children. When they cannot do it then the local community is responsible. When the local community cannot handle it, it is up to the county and then the State, and lastly it is up to Uncle Sam to be responsible for feeding the children of this Nation. With that as a basis of my opposition to this bill, I wish to state that I conducted a school-lunch program, that we did give free lunches, that we did provide free milk for undernourished children, but we did it all at the expense of the local community by raising the money locally, by putting on school programs to raise the money to give free milk to those children whose parents could not afford to do it.[27]

Federal involvement in school lunch programs, according to this view, was to be reserved for emergencies only; any permanent development should occur at the local and state levels.

Evidence suggested, however, that at least some areas still relied heavily on federal aid. Frank Washam, director of lunchrooms of the Chicago Board of Education and president of the National School Cafeteria Association, reported a 403 percent increase in milk consumption at Chicago high schools when federal investment reduced the price of a half pint of milk from five cents to one cent.[28] War Food Administrator Marvin Jones claimed that "lack of a permanent program of Federal assistance has deterred many State governments from actively entering into the school-lunch program."[29] Despite higher wages, many children still could not afford adequate food, and many schools lacked the money, the resources, or the skilled labor to begin meal programs.

The conservative argument from tradition was related to trepidation over the financial advisability of federal investment in school lunch programs. With the U.S. government a record $300 billion in debt at the end of the war, concern about deficit spending was not unwarranted. However, the minuscule appropriations connected with school lunch legislation were too small to make any significant difference in the federal budget, and so the argument for curtailing spending was one of principle rather than pragmatism. Proponents of federal involvement ridiculed the fiscal responsibility position as at best disingenuous and at worst willfully callous. "Huge sums are appropriated . . . to eradicate diseases of livestock," Wisconsin representative Andrew Biemiller said, trotting out a popular hobby horse, "but certainly simple justice and common sense should tell us that if we can afford large sums to protect livestock we can spend $50,000,000 to insure a sound, healthy rising generation."[30] Biemiller, a socialist and liberal leader, urged Congress to regard access to food as a human right, criticizing the conservative platform of traditional order and fiscal responsibility. Others pointed out the absurdity of feeding children overseas but not at home. "After all is said and done," Vermont representative Charles Plumley told his colleagues, "we should not spend billions to feed people and children in devastated areas while we let our own children starve."[31] Indeed, Congress approved $2.7 billion in food aid for Europe during the war but routinely quibbled over appropriations as little as $50 million per year to subsidize the feeding of American children.[32]

Conservatives also relied on the equivalence of "social welfare" with "socialism," much as they had for decades, as a justification to reduce not only federal expenditures but federal involvement. In response, Flannagan argued that "the dictator nations exist upon hungry bodies and befuddled minds," while others pointed out that similar accusations of socialism were levied against free public education, resource conservation, unemployment insurance, old-age pensions, the WPA, and numerous other beloved federal programs.[33] "In my opinion," Russell said, addressing the Senate, "a school child who has a good bowl of hot soup and glass of sweet milk for his lunch will be much more likely to be able to resist communism or socialism than would one who had for his lunch a hard biscuit which had been baked the day before and which he had brought with him to school in a tin can."[34] Massachusetts representative John McCormack warned the House that "the quickest road to communism and radicalism is for those entrusted with the responsibility, care, and conduct of Government, to fail to recognize that the first obligation of government is to bring justice to its people, and to forget those who are underprivileged."[35]

Encouraged by broad support, Ellender and Russell submitted an amended bill (S. 962) to the Senate in May of 1945, in which they combined elements of the Russell Bill and the Smith-Ellender Bill. Flannagan introduced a similar version of the bill (H.R. 3370) to the House one month later.[36] The amended school lunch bill had two titles: Title I allocated $100 million annually to the USDA for distribution of both surplus foods and matching grants for food purchases; Title II assigned $15 million annually to the U.S. Bureau of Education for distribution to state education authorities "to establish, maintain, operate, and expand school-lunch programs, to provide related nutrition education, and to provide and train technical and supervisory personnel and to provide equipment and facilities for such programs."[37]

The most notable concession in this compromise was that the USDA received the bulk of the funding, putting an emphasis on surplus disposal over public health nutrition or nutrition education. Russell himself refused to support school lunch legislation if the meals were not connected to the reduction of agricultural surpluses, and this was a widely held position both in Congress and in the leadership of the USDA.[38] The farm lobby was a powerful one, and farm organizations such as the American Farm Bureau Federation, the National Grange, the National Council of Farmer Cooperatives, and the National Cooperative Milk Producers Federation urged passage of the bill in large part because "control of the program rests in the hands of the Secretary of Agriculture."[39] In fact, this was one of the only pieces of federal legislation to be endorsed by every major farm organization.

Tension between public health nutrition and agricultural surplus disposal involved more than competing interests. The level of prioritization assigned to each of these disparate functions would establish the primary purpose of the legislation itself. Was the federal school lunch program to be one of surplus disposal that happened to provide nutritious food for schoolchildren, or one of public health nutrition that happened to provide an outlet for excess foods? This distinction was by no means trivial, as it would determine the balance struck not only between the needs of consumers and producers but also between the promotion of health and the protection of wealth.

The educational aspects of the school lunch bill proved to be one of the most contentious issues, but they were also a part of the legislation that could help define the school lunch bill as primarily a health act. As Ellender put it:

> The school lunch, properly directed, becomes an activity through which children learn some of the most important lessons of life; namely, the production, conservation, purchase, preparation, serving, and consuming of foods. But to accomplish these purposes the school lunch must become an integrated part of the entire school program. It must be managed by technically trained supervisors who have the ability not only to put the funds provided to most effective use but to help all the children to secure from the school lunch program maximum benefits both nutritionally and educationally.[40]

Without an educational component, along with careful nutritional supervision, school meals were at best a palliative measure. Since the turn of the century, physicians and nutritionists had argued that the biggest public health gains would come from changes made to children's diets *outside* of school; although the meal served at lunchtime could and did improve health, behavior, and academic performance, school lunches represented at best only five of a child's (ideally) twenty-one meals each week.

Title II of the school lunch bill came under concerted attack from conservative House Republicans. "[This act] means eventual Federal control of the school systems of the country," Ohio representative Cliff Clevenger warned. "If you participate in this thing you will find that under title II you have lost control of your free public-school system."[41] Minnesota representative August Andresen, a senior member of the House Committee on Agriculture, opposed Title II because it would "tell the people what they have to eat" and "create another agency in Washington to add to hundreds of agencies now existing that are eating out of the taxpayers' pocketbook."[42] One representative even went so far as to call the U.S. Bureau of Education "a menace to the public school system."[43] Despite the fact that the bill authorized the bureau only to apportion money—not to set state education policy nor to interfere in any way with school operations—resistance to Title II was widespread in Congress. Even southern Democrats, most of whom were staunch supporters of school lunch legislation, worried about the erosion of states' rights seemingly implicit in the legislation. When Andresen moved to strike Title II from the House bill entirely, the measure passed by a two-to-one margin.[44]

Senator Robert Taft of Ohio, a prominent opponent of the New Deal and leading member of the conservative coalition, likewise called for the removal of Title II from the Senate bill. "To set up a new Federal control over the diet and food of the people of this country," he argued, "seems to me to go beyond anything we have done heretofore and beyond the existing school-lunch program." But when the vote on whether to strike Title II was taken, the Senate elected to retain it by a two-to-one margin and sent the bill back to the House, which refused to budge, effectively stalling the bill.[45]

The debate over the so-called federalization of public education, however, was only part of the issue for which school lunches had become a prominent context. Politicians on both sides of the aisle and from all parts of the country regarded school lunch legislation as a proxy battlefield in the growing fight over school segregation and civil rights. *Plessy v. Ferguson*, the 1896 Supreme Court decision that legalized segregation as long as the facilities were "separate but equal," had effectively legitimized racial discrimination. In the 1920s, the National Association for the Advancement of Colored People (NAACP) showed that although schools in the South were invariably separate, they were anything but equal. Georgia schools, for example, spent $36.29 for each white child but only $4.59 for each black child, and black teachers earned half what white teachers earned. Even in North Carolina, the southern state that came closest to economic parity, education authorities spent more on white pupils, and the average salary of black teachers was two-thirds that of white teachers.[46] This kind of racism was most common in the South, but numerous other states, including Arizona, California, New Jersey, and Pennsylvania, maintained racially segregated schools.

In addition, the hardships of the Depression were not equally distributed. More than two-thirds of black cotton growers in the early 1930s made no profit, either breaking even or plunging further into debt. To make matters worse, urban jobs traditionally filled by blacks— street cleaning, garbage removal, domestic service, cooking, and elevator operation—were increasingly given to unemployed whites. By 1932, more than half of the black workers in southern cities were unemployed, and those in northern cities fared little better; unemployment rates were more than 40 percent in Chicago, Detroit, and New York City, and more than 50 percent in Philadelphia. Blacks also received considerably less state relief than whites, particularly in the South, where states granted the lowest unemployment benefits in the nation.[47] Although health had improved considerably in the early twentieth century—between 1900 and 1930, average life expectancy nationwide rose from 47.3 years to 59.7 years, and the gross mortality rate fell from 17.6 per 1,000 to 11.9 per 1,000, a 33 percent reduction—the average life expectancy at birth of a black infant was still more than ten years shorter than for whites, and both total mortality and infant mortality rates were markedly higher.[48]

Early drafts of the school lunch bill contained surprisingly progressive language with respect to race, especially considering the racist views of the primary architects. No Title I funds could "be paid or disbursed to any State or school if, in carrying out its functions under this title, it makes any discrimination because of race, creed, color, or national origin of children or between types of schools or, with respect to a State which maintains separate schools for minority and for majority races, it discriminates between such schools on this account."[49] Title II stipulated that "if the State maintains separate schools for minority and majority races, provisions shall be contained [in the 'State plan for the administration of school-lunch programs'] necessary to assure a just and equitable distribution of the funds under this title for the benefit of such minority races."[50] The House Committee on Agriculture removed this language from the bill on the grounds that it was "unnecessary," as even Flannagan himself had testified that "no discrimination has been made heretofore in the [federal] program with respect to race or color or creed."[51] This was, perhaps, disingenuous, as the federal government neither defined discrimination in this context nor investigated it in any way. Indeed, the fact that schools had essentially to establish a lunch program and then request federal reimbursement made it virtually impossible for resource-poor schools to do so.

When Adam Clayton Powell—one of only two black members of Congress at a time when federal buildings still had segregated facilities—suggested that the House amend the bill back to its original state, the proposition was thoroughly defeated. Georgia representative Malcolm Tarver argued that such language would not improve the federal school lunch program and would, in fact, reduce support for it.

> I have never been advised by anyone of any discrimination anywhere in the United States in the administration of the program, on account of race, color, creed, or any other condition of that type. . . . I regret very much to see injected into the subject matter of this bill something which I believe is entirely unnecessary to consider and which, if it is adopted, will not in any way affect the administration of the school-lunch program as it is at present being carried on. It seems to me the only effect of adopting this amendment would be to alienate some votes that otherwise might be cast for approval of the pending bill. . . . I can see no objection to the amendment, although I think it is a trouble-making amendment which may endanger enactment of the bill, and I shall vote against it.[52]

Although there was no evidence of overt racial discrimination during the ten years in which the federal government had operated school lunch programs, neither was there an equitable distribution of federal resources.

In Mississippi, for example, the WPA provided labor for school meal programs in 839 schools for whites and only 164 schools for blacks, serving lunches to approximately 75,000 children in 1936.[53] The population of Mississippi was more than half black, but only 16 percent of the schools with federal lunch programs served black children. Although this was the first time that any of the state's black schools received government support for meals, white children as a whole clearly benefited more than black children from federal investment. Such inequality was a form of discrimination not acknowledged as such in federal statistics, and so the Powell amendment was an attempt to require that states rectify these structural inequities proactively in order to receive federal funds.

While Tarver opposed the amendment ostensibly on the basis of political compromise, in reality, southern politicians feared that it would provide a precedent for the federal government to equate segregation itself with discrimination; Congress would, according to this view, effectively dismantle legalized segregation because the antidiscrimination clause in federal school lunch legislation would create a new legal basis for regarding "separate but equal" as inherently discriminatory. In the face of heavy opposition, Powell withdrew his amendment from consideration without even putting it to a vote.[54] Civil rights reformers were unwilling to sacrifice funding for school meals in order to challenge racial inequities.

While it is likely that school meal programs were implemented in at least some black schools prior to federal involvement, documentation of such programs does not seem to have survived. Discussions of race with respect to school meals, as chapter 3 explores, tended in the early twentieth century to focus on the dietary needs of various ethnic and national groups, especially the Irish, Italians, and Jews. Yet even in these cases, most programs ceased to cater specifically to different needs by the 1920s, offering instead fairly standardized menus. Thus it is perhaps surprising that race even came up in the congressional debates over school meals, as it had not been a significant part of school foodservice discussions for some two decades by that time. It is even more surprising that Russell and Ellender would actively promote legislation that provided even weak support for civil rights. While it is difficult to do more than speculate as to the reasons for these inconsistencies, it is likely that the situation of school meals at the intersection of health, education, and social welfare, and within an ongoing debate over the proper distribution of rights and responsibilities for children's well-being, made school meals a useful context for negotiating national policy on a range of issues, even those not previously prominent in national discussions.

Indeed, the public health aspects of the school lunch bill, though not as controversial as the education or civil rights elements, provoked debate as well. Proponents of the bill advocated its importance, even its necessity, in the national public health infrastructure. "Because it is health insurance," Wisconsin representative La Vern Dilweg stated, "it is expected every child in America will soon receive the benefit of school lunches."[55] Many felt that nutrition was the best preventive approach that could be taken against infectious diseases and acquired disability. "Since our doctors are not yet able to provide a serum, or a vaccine, or an anti-toxin against every disease and infection," argued Pennsylvania representative Augustine Kelley, chair of the House Subcommittee on Aid to the Physically Handicapped, "[good food] is the best protection we know against infectious diseases, which bring in their wake the damaged vision, the damaged ears, and the damaged hearts which may disable for life."[56] A nutrition vaccination, proponents argued, could protect children from disease better than almost any other medical intervention.

Many of the bill's opponents continued to argue from tradition—with an often explicit critique of scientific and medical expertise—that the federal government was not well suited for a role in public health nutrition. It was a question of "whether or not the mothers of America . . . or the bureaucrats who work in these bureaus know more about how to feed the children," Ohio representative Frederick Smith argued. "So far as I am concerned, I would rather have the mothers in my community decide that they are going to give these children milk and vegetables and meat and fruit than to have some bureaucrat come in from a distance and determine what they shall have to eat."[57] This not only affirmed the traditional chain of responsibility—from mothers to local authorities to the state and finally to the federal government—but also challenged the expertise of nutrition science itself. Of course, historically it had been women and mothers who most supported the efforts of schools to provide meals for children as a health measure. Regardless, conservatives used mothers as a foil, construing the school lunch bill as an attack on the home. "Perhaps our poor mothers . . . did the best with what they had," Michigan representative Clare Hoffman chastised his colleagues. "Are you ashamed of what your mother did for you or what your dad did when he applied the little old barrel stave out in the woodshed? Sometimes I think he did not use it often enough on some of us."[58]

Others opposed the bill from a position of antagonism to federally provided health care. North Carolina senator Harold Cooley asked why, if the government were to feed children for free, it should not also "provide medical care and dental care and hospitalization for all poor children."[59] Opposition to "socialized" medicine—from both physicians and politicians—had been pronounced since World War I and had successfully defeated nearly all attempts to legislate mandatory health insurance or otherwise involve the federal government in the provision of healthcare.

During the spring of 1946, Congress ultimately formed a bicameral committee to draft a school lunch bill that addressed the desires and concerns expressed during the two years of debate that had surrounded the initiative. Six members of the House Committee on Agriculture and five members of the Senate Committee on Agriculture and Forestry composed a bill that would appease the legislation's detractors, and thus pass, but the resulting bill was a mere shadow of its forerunners.[60]

The most significant change the committee made was to remove Title II from the bill. In exchange for this concession to the House, the committee reduced the cap on the ratio of state matching funds from four-to-one to three-to-one and inserted language into the bill allowing funds disbursed by the secretary of agriculture, up to $10 million per year, to be used for "nonfood assistance," including "the cost of processing, distributing, transporting, storing, or handling [foods]."[61] In addition to eliminating Title II, the committee scrubbed all references to nutrition education from the bill and added language to specifically forbid federal involvement in education: "In carrying out the provisions of this Act, neither the Secretary [of Agriculture] nor the State shall impose any requirement with respect to teaching personnel, curriculum, instruction, methods of instruction, and materials of instruction in any school."[62] This effectively eliminated any federal support for nutrition education, without which there was neither a requirement nor an incentive for states to develop or provide nutrition education in tandem with school meals. More than anything else, this made the bill primarily a price-support measure for agriculture and only incidentally a nutrition program for children.

The revised bill was not a measure of "health insurance," as Dilweg had advocated. Nor was "the big thing—the controlling thing in the program," as Flannagan told a CBS Radio audience, "furnishing underprivileged and undernourished American boys and girls a wholesome, nutritious meal, so they will develop mentally and physically into strong American men and women."[63] Rather, it became a measure of "national security."[64] National security could be interpreted in a political or military context, in which the health of (future) citizens and soldiers is a key component, or in the context of food security, in which the regulation of agriculture is a key component, but in neither case does the phrase indicate that the bill was primarily a health bill. In fact, the revised bill made virtually no health provisions, save that the meals served must "meet minimum nutritional requirements," which were to be determined by the USDA.[65]

The changes made to the school lunch bill, though they rendered its most progressive elements inert, also ensured that it would pass. Stripped of protections for civil rights, support for nutrition education, and a clear prioritization of children's health, it was passed by Congress in May, and President Harry Truman signed the National School Lunch Act into law on 4 June 1946, the month when the temporary school lunch measures expired.[66]

The National School Lunch Act established a number of requirements for states to receive federal money for school lunch programs. It required schools to sell lunches on a nonprofit basis, to make them available at reduced cost or free to impoverished children "without physical segregation . . . or other discrimination," to sell only lunches that met "minimum nutrition requirements," to utilize surplus commodities "insofar as practicable," and to report their expenditures and receipts to state education authorities.[67] In return, the federal government would allocate each year's apportionment to state education authorities according to the number of school children (i.e., children aged 5–17) in each state. Until 1950, the government would match state investments dollar for dollar; after 1950, states would receive $1.00 for every $1.50 they invested, and after 1955 $1.00 for every $3.00. In states where the per capita income was below the national average, the matching requirement would be reduced by the same percentage as the difference between the state's mean income and the U.S. mean income.[68]

The National School Lunch Act thus represented both an unparalleled triumph and a miserable failure. On one hand, reform-minded physicians, nutritionists, politicians, teachers, and mothers secured a permanent foundation for school meal programs. More than four decades of development had transformed school lunches from a grassroots, community-based initiative into a national food assistance program with steady funding. Never before had the federal government become directly involved in the conduct of schooling, and the NSLP soon became the nation's most extensive national health program for school-aged children. The farm bloc gained federal protection from overproduction and some measure of price control; southern Democrats brought federal money into their states without relinquishing the right to control its expenditure, maintaining the racially segregated status quo; for the first time, schools could rely on permanent federal support to ensure that children would be able to handle the rigors of education; and health authorities brought federal attention, however weak, to the problem of public health nutrition.

On the other hand, the National School Lunch Act was itself a rather malnourished health initiative. The historian Susan Levine has argued that passage of the National School Lunch Act resulted from a number of "uneasy compromise[s]," between conservative southern Democrats and northern New Deal liberals, between the farm bloc and social welfare advocates, between nutritionists and agricultural economists, and between civil rights crusaders and segregationists.[69] In fact, the National School Lunch Act required virtually no compromises from the farm bloc or from segregationists, while the interests of health authorities, nutritionists, and civil rights activists were virtually absent from the legislation. It was a compromise only in the sense that some goals were entirely compromised to ensure passage of the bill, but it was in many respects a Pyrrhic victory.

The elimination of Title II and removal of all support for nutrition education was a significant blow to those pursuing school lunch legislation in order to promote public health nutrition. Nutritionists and health authorities seemed resigned to take whatever they could get, even if it meant suborning children's nutrition to agricultural protection. Bessie West, president of the American Dietetic Association, urged Congress to pass the bill despite her organization's belief that it "should make provision for proper supervision and adequate nutritional education."[70] Indeed, the bill received endorsements from virtually all health and nutrition organizations, who tacitly took a something-is-better-than-nothing approach.[71] Not only was nutrition education absent from the legislation, but the NSLP also proved unable even to provide nutritious meals. Well into the twenty-first century, as numerous scholars and journalists have shown, most federally subsidized school meals were unappetizing and nutritionally poor, and the most needy and disadvantaged children were the least likely to benefit from the program.[72]

Civil rights promoters also failed to secure legislation that would prevent racial discrimination. Although the National School Lunch Act included a clause to ensure "a just and equitable distribution . . . for the benefit of such minority races," all reference to racial discrimination was removed.[73] The remaining language basically reiterated the "separate but equal" policy by which many states legally maintained stark racial divisions. Without a stated enforcement policy, blacks and other racial minorities remained the victims of pervasive neglect and overt discrimination.

As late as the 1970s, significant racial disparities were still common. In Las Vegas, "the city of all-you-can-eat, forty-nine-cent buffets," poor black children were not getting breakfasts or lunches at school. Although Clark County received federal money to provide free meals, school administrators claimed that Westside schools did not have adequate kitchen equipment and "the district could not afford to upgrade them," something that did not prevent the serving of hot meals at white schools with comparable facilities. Clark County served fewer than 300 meals in a district with 8,000 children living on public assistance. Furthermore, "school administrators in at least a dozen cities were using federal lunch moneys to provide hot lunches in affluent districts while providing inexpensive cold lunches in poor neighborhoods," something that affected racial minorities disproportionately.[74] Experiences such as these spawned the Right to Lunch movement in the late 1960s and early 1970s; twenty years after the passage of the National School Lunch Act, the lack of antidiscrimination language was continuing to have profound effects on the implementation of federally supported school meals.

The NSLP, ostensibly the longest-running and most extensive children's health program in U.S. history, ultimately contained no educational component, only the most minimal nutrition standards, no specific health agenda, no provision for training or supervision, and nothing to prevent discrimination, racial or otherwise. Despite its stated goal "to safeguard the health and well-being of the Nation's children and to encourage the domestic consumption of nutritious agricultural commodities and other food," the NSLP, as it was conceived in 1946 and as it was implemented for most of its history, was ultimately an agricultural protection measure far more than a nutrition education or children's health initiative.

Epilogue

> When, gentlemen, our schools have taken hold of this subject [of
> nutrition] and taught its principles, . . . then will you and I not be
> called to witness the harrowing spectacle of emaciated and starved
> infants in the arms of loving and devoted mothers whose careworn
> faces tell of sleepless weeks and exhausted bodies, whose eager
> eyes watch our every move and expression, and whose questions
> bespeak their anxiety and mental suffering. . . . This subject, gentle-
> men, lies at the very foundation of our boasted humanity.
> —Charles Douglas, addressing the Detroit Medical
> and Library Association, 1899[1]

In 1945, with passage of the National School Lunch Act imminent,
Surgeon General Thomas Parran remarked that "one important incidental result of such a school-lunch program will be to encourage the
consumption and production of nutritionally useful foods."[2] His use
of the term "incidental" is telling, as these were not specific aims for
which policies were established or funding committed. At best, such
effects on production and consumption would be the side effects of a
program ultimately more focused on agricultural economics and food
security than on children's nutritional health and education. Health
and education authorities, among them Parran himself, had pushed
for more extensive school meal legislation, but most of their goals—
including comprehensive food and nutrition education, antidiscrimination policies, a broad nutrition health agenda, and optimal (rather
than minimal) nutrition standards—went unrealized. Not only did
Parran's prediction prove wrong, but the trend in the second half of
the twentieth century moved in the opposite direction: both production and consumption arguably became less "nutritionally useful," not
more. There is no conclusive evidence from the twentieth century that
the NSLP caused (or even encouraged) children to eat more healthful
foods, and the school as a market stimulated no significant changes in

agricultural production. This is unsurprising, as one of the core functions of the NSLP was to absorb surplus foods, thus sheltering producers from market variability and reducing the need to adapt production in response to demand.

Neither has children's desire for junk food diminished. The girl who today eats "chips, soda, maybe a chocolate ice cream taco" for lunch because, she explains, "that's all I like to eat" is not very different from the boy of her great-great-grandparents' generation who ate a dozen crullers at lunchtime despite it being "bad for the health."[3] And malnutrition remains a central concern in contemporary public health, perhaps *the* central concern as tobacco use has continued to decline. U.S. Surgeon General David Satcher estimated in 2001 that "13 percent of children and adolescents were overweight," and he cautioned that "overweight and obesity may soon cause as much preventable disease and death as cigarette smoking."[4] This echoed Parran's own concerns about malnourishment from six decades earlier: "Something like 9,000,000 school children are not getting a diet adequate for health and well-being," he wrote in 1942. "And malnutrition is our greatest producer of ill health."[5] As an education problem and as a health problem, malnourishment abides. Just one year after Surgeon General Satcher released his report, researchers at the RAND Corporation deemed the health risks associated with obesity to be worse than those associated with smoking, drinking, or poverty.[6]

After reading this book, one may be forgiven for feeling that the past is repeating itself. Against the backdrop of a national nutrition health crisis (now centered around pervasive overweight rather than underweight) and continuing concern about the impact of socioeconomic inequity on access to nutritious foods, new voices and movements have emerged that bear striking similarity to those of the early twentieth century. Exposés such as Eric Schlosser's *Fast Food Nation* (2001), Morgan Spurlock's *Super Size Me* (2004), and Michael Pollan's *The Omnivore's Dilemma* (2006) have once again focused national attention on the relationships between food, industry, socioeconomic status, and health, much as Robert Hunter's *Poverty* (1904), Upton Sinclair's *The Jungle* (1906), and John Spargo's *Underfed Schoolchildren* (1906) did at the turn of the twentieth century.[7] Similarly, school gardens, farm-to-school programs, ethnically tailored menus, anti-junk-food policies, and other Progressive Era wheels are being reinvented. And once again, politicians and military leaders are characterizing malnourishment as a significant threat to national security, arguing that nutritional improvement is critical for the future well-being of the nation.[8]

In 2002, for example, Oakland, California, became one of the first big cities to eliminate junk foods from schools. The district, which educates more than 50,000 children, banned the sale of candy, caffeinated drinks, and other unhealthful foods on school grounds.[9] The Institute of Medicine, which advises Congress on issues of science and health, has consistently advocated this as a national policy recommendation, and many reformers called for legislative action to enforce it.[10] But these are not new concerns; such attempts were also common a century ago. The prominent pediatrician and nutritionist Lulu Hunt Peters lobbied to ban candy from schools in Boston in the early twentieth century. The 1930 White House Conference on Child Health and Protection advised that "the sale of candy in the lunchroom should be limited. Candy should never be sold to children who have not had a 'good lunch' and should never be displayed in ways and quantities beyond the average child's powers of resistance."[11] Much as early school meal programs struggled to overcome the allure that candy and fast food had for children, today's debates over the place of such foods in schools pit public health nutrition against children's preferences and economic incentives. In banning junk foods, Oakland lost $650,000 per year in revenue, money that funded athletic programs, camping trips, and other healthful activities.[12] In this, too, there are echoes of the past: "I can't let you stop my Christmas candy sales," an elementary school principal told the school's nutrition worker in the 1920s, "for that's my only source of income for pictures and all our extras." Candy sales, another said, brought in "very desirable dollars."[13] Then as now, schools' economic incentives and the cultivation of healthy pupils were not well aligned.

Many schools now are also trying to change the lunch menu itself, enticing children to eat healthier food by appealing to the tastes of common ethnic or national groups. MS 137 in Queens, New York, for example, must feed nearly 2,000 students a day. The school, like many others in New York City, is a melting pot. Class materials are available in eight languages because many of the students come from Guyanese, Dominican, and Bengali families. Trying to tempt children away from fast food, the school has added curry to the lunch menu. The curry must be made with approved ingredients—"frozen pre-roasted commodity chicken parts, jarred chopped garlic, and a generic curry powder"—but dishes also include fresh onions, green peppers, and celery. "The kids love this curry," the school's lunchroom director told the *New York Times*. "It makes them feel comforted and cared for, which is what we want to do." Serving ethnic foods in schools, as was common in many early meal programs, today faces challenges beyond the restricted ingredients available. Of the 1,385 school kitchens in New York City, only half have equipment that allows cooking over an open flame. In many of those that do have such fixtures, "aging ovens sometimes don't heat properly, equipment is hidden away in storage rooms or broken, and the staff isn't trained to do much more than steam frozen vegetables, dig ravioli out of a six-pound can, or heat frozen chicken patties in a convection oven." In fact, more than 80 percent of American school districts cook fewer than half of their entrees from scratch.[14]

Schools are attempting not only to reform menus but also to reform the ingredients themselves. School gardens, farm-to-school programs, and local purchasing arrangements are attempts to replace heavily processed foods, like most of the surplus commodities available through the NSLP, with fresh or minimally processed, locally produced foods. The state of California, for instance, passed an initiative in 2002 to encourage the planting and maintenance of a garden in every school. Thousands of schools now have gardens, which teachers utilize in lessons on nutrition, agriculture, language arts, mathematics, and physical activity. Many school gardens supply edible produce, and studies have shown that they lead to higher vegetable consumption when supplemented with classroom instruction.[15] Most schools cannot rely on gardens for produce throughout the school year, due in part to inclement weather and in part to space constraints, but many schools are also pursuing partnerships with local farms to supply raw materials for children's lunches.

In this most recent iteration of the farm-to-school model, nearly 10,000 schools in forty-seven states were engaged in some sort of direct purchasing arrangement with local producers as of 2011. Like the cooperative cafeterias that emerged in rural areas, particularly during the Great Depression, farm-to-school programs promote the use of school meals to bridge the health interests of local children and the economic interests of local farmers. Unlike the National School Lunch Act, which created virtually no reciprocal relationship between producers and consumers, farm-to-school programs may help to achieve the agricultural reforms that Surgeon General Parran hoped would result from a national meal program, for they place schools and farms on relatively equal footing in their economic interactions. Such programs, however, still face competition from lunch trucks and other food vendors operating outside schools. Students often spend as much or more on junk foods outside of school because they don't like the meals served in the cafeteria, where, as one student put it, "they have, like, fruits and vegetables."[16]

This recent activism has begun to stimulate change, not only in isolated cases but nationally as well, and it is likely that the NSLP will undergo considerable restructuring in the coming years. The Healthy, Hunger-Free Kids Act, which was passed in 2010 and implemented in 2012, has already introduced sweeping changes to national policies surrounding children's nutrition, and in particular to the NSLP. The implementation of the act's provisions has instigated one of the most extensive debates in U.S. history over children's nutrition and the role of the school in children's health, but it has also introduced the most significant structural changes to the NSLP since it began in 1947.

For the first time, national legislation has coupled school meal provision with targeted health and nutrition directives, something for which reformers in the early twentieth century fought unsuccessfully. In addition to increasing federal funding for school meals, the act authorizes schools to provide free meals to all students based on community eligibility if at least 40 percent of attending students would qualify for free meals individually. For the first time, free meals are widely available for those who need them most. In order to receive continued federal support, states must conduct regular reviews of the nutritional content of school meals, and participating schools must establish a "wellness policy" that includes nutritional health and physical fitness. In addition, all foods not included in the federally subsidized meals but sold on school grounds, including snacks and beverages dispensed from vending machines, must conform to nutrition standards established by the USDA.[17] In other words, the Healthy, Hunger-Free Kids Act is in many ways the legislation that early reformers hoped, but ultimately failed, to enact.

Yet even with these changes, there are fundamental obstacles that continue to hinder the development of comprehensive school meal programs. Decades of airplane-style meals, which require little more than reheating, have deskilled the labor force, removed cooking equipment from school kitchens, and supported a powerful industry that has profited on the preparation, distribution, and serving of such meals.[18] In addition, it remains difficult to provide unequivocal data on hunger and malnourishment, and on the impact of school meals on children's nutritional health. Unlike public health programs developed to reduce tobacco use, which can use sales as a proxy for consumption, the distribution of meals to children is a poor metric for nutritional intake. If children throw away some of the food they receive, it alters the program's efficacy, but it is virtually impossible to measure with any reliability the actual consumption of food, let alone how it affects children's health and well-being. And despite initiatives like school gardens and farm-to-school programs, most schools remain heavily dependent on surplus commodities and precooked meals designed to meet federal standards, ensuring that children continue to receive foods that few find appetizing. As if all of this were not enough, many students have only twenty minutes for lunch, including the time it takes to get to the cafeteria, wait in line for food, and eat.

The Healthy, Hunger-Free Kids Act has made many positive changes to what had been an increasingly moribund health and welfare program, but the NSLP is still a far cry from the systemic, holistic intervention envisioned by those who created the country's first school meal programs. While children and the schools that educate them face different problems today than a century ago, the need for supplemental feeding and nutritional improvement is no less pressing, and public support for school meals no less strong. Yet history suggests that without development of a system that integrates eating and learning, that values skilled labor and community involvement, and that privileges children's health over agricultural protection, malnourishment will continue to be "our greatest producer of ill health."

Acknowledgments

Clifford Ashley, who completed a thousand-page tome on the tying of knots in 1944, wrote in his introduction that "the urge to write a book is nowadays accepted as ample excuse for almost any delinquency." This book, however, is about lunches, and although I consumed some two thousand of them while researching and writing it, the most delinquent thing I had occasion to do was omit a full serving of vegetables. My *next* book will be about robot space pirates. Or pie.

Setting aside the deplorable absence of opportunities for delinquency, this project benefited from the time and resources of numerous individuals and institutions. Judy Leavitt and Rima Apple read multiple drafts, and their insights made the manuscript much, much better. I am also indebted to Peter Mickulas at Rutgers University Press, whose enthusiasm for the project remained unwavering, and to the two reviewers who read the manuscript and offered criticisms that were spot on. David Williamson Shaffer has been a fantastic writing partner, and my writing is better for having worked on papers and grants with him.

I was fortunate enough to receive financial support from the Robert Wood Johnson Foundation Health and Society Scholars Program, the State of the Art Conference on Home Economics at the University of Georgia, the University of Wisconsin Institute for Research in the Humanities, and the Department of the History of Science and Department of Medical History and Bioethics at the University of Wisconsin–Madison. No delinquencies were bankrolled by these institutions, though not for lack of trying. Of course, the conclusions presented in this book are mine alone, and may not (yet) reflect the views of the funding agencies, their partners, or their subsidiaries.

The research for this book turned out to be far more challenging than expected. Apparently few of the people who lived at the beginning of the last century anticipated my need for detailed and accurate accounts of early school meal initiatives. Some of them did anticipate my needs (thanks!), but in many cases their courtesy was rudely negated by floods, fires, and other record-destroying calamities. It is entirely possible that my bloodline is cursed. Be that as it may, I am deeply indebted to the many librarians and archivists who answered questions and helped me track down materials that do still exist, including staff at Butler Library (Columbia University); the Chicago Public Library; Ebling Health Sciences Library (University of Wisconsin–Madison); the Herbert Hoover Presidential Library; the Kansas City Public Library; the Library of Congress; the National Agricultural Library; the National Archives; the National Library of Medicine; the New York Academy of Medicine; the New York Public Library; the Enoch Pratt Free Library; the Regenstein Library (University of Chicago); the Richard B. Russell Library for Political Research and Studies (University of Georgia); the St. Louis Public Library; the University of Illinois, Chicago, University Library; the University of Wisconsin Archives; and the Wisconsin State Historical Society. And those are only the libraries and archives I visited in meatspace. I must have visited at least ten times as many cybraries and digital archives, far too many to list here, but I especially want to thank the army of laborers who scanned and catalogued resources that I could not have accessed otherwise. Their work made mine possible.

Now, I wasn't entirely honest about the lack of opportunity for delinquency. As a reward for having read the acknowledgments section, know that there are several copies of this very book in which is secreted a golden ticket, good for one reasonably priced, nutritionally adequate lunch with the author. Airfare and accommodations are not included, but hey, free lunch!

Notes

Introduction

1. Quoted in Albertina Bechmann, "The First Penny Lunch," *Journal of Home Economics* 25, no. 9 (1933): 762.
2. *Fed up with Lunch: The School Lunch Project*, http://fedupwithschool lunch.blogspot.com/, accessed 8 March 2011. Mrs. Q later revealed her identity and published a book about her experiences: Sarah Wu, *Fed Up with Lunch: The School Lunch Project: How One Anonymous Teacher Revealed the Truth about School Lunches—And How We Can Change Them!* (San Francisco: Chronicle Books, 2011).
3. William Christeson, Amy Dawson Taggart, and Soren Messner-Zidell, *Too Fat to Fight* (Washington, DC: Mission: Readiness, 2010), 3; *The Surgeon General's Vision for a Healthy and Fit Nation* (Washington, DC: U.S. Department of Health and Human Services, 2010), 1.
4. Data obtained from the USDA Food and Nutrition Service: http:// www.fns.usda.gov/cnd/governance/notices/naps/NAPs10–11.pdf.
5. Healthy, Hunger-Free Kids Act, Pub. L. 111–296, 111th Congress, 2nd Session (13 December 2010), §§ 204, 208.
6. Nicholas Confessore, "How School Lunch Became the Latest Political Battleground," *New York Times Magazine*, 7 October 2014.
7. *National School Lunch Program Fact Sheet* (Washington, DC: U.S. Department of Agriculture, 2013), http://www.fns.usda.gov/sites/default /files/NSLPFactSheet.pdf.
8. Confessore, "How School Lunch Became the Latest Political Battleground."
9. Susan Levine, *School Lunch Politics: The Surprising History of America's Favorite Welfare Program* (Princeton: Princeton University Press, 2008), 2.
10. The most extensive histories of school meals in the United States are Levine, *School Lunch Politics* and Gordon W. Gunderson, *The National School Lunch Program: Background and Development* (New York: Nova Science Publishers, 2003). A notable exception to the focus on the NSLP is William J. Reese, "After Bread, Education: Nutrition and Urban School Children, 1890–1920," *Teachers College Record* 81, no. 4 (1980): 496–525.
11. I have been able to identify forty-six U.S. cities that were administering meal programs by 1913: Albany (NY), Amherst (MA), Boston (MA), Buffalo (NY), Chicago (IL), Cincinnati (OH), Cleveland (OH), Columbus (OH), Dallas (TX), Denver (CO), Eau Claire (WI), Erie (PA), Fairhaven (?),

Grand Rapids (MI), Greenfield (MA), Hartford (CT), Houston (TX), India-
napolis (IN), Kansas City (MO), Logansville (PA), Los Angeles (CA), Louis-
ville (KY), Manayunk (PA), McKeesport (PA), Memphis (TN), Mill Valley
(NY), Milwaukee (WI), Montpelier (VT), Muskegon (MI), New Haven (CT),
New Orleans (LA), Newtonville (MA), New York City (NY), Omaha (NE),
Philadelphia (PA), Pittsburgh (PA), Providence (RI), Rochester (NY), St.
Louis (MO), St. Paul (MN), Seattle (WA), Toledo (OH), Utica (NY), Wash-
ington, DC, Wayne (PA), and Westford (MA).

12. Irene C. Harrington, "The High-School Lunch: Its Financial, Admin-
    istrative, and Educational Policies," *Journal of Home Economics* 16, no. 11
    (1924): 625.

13. The figure given is in unadjusted dollars. S. K. Hargis, "The School as
    a Market for Food Products," *American Food Journal* 21, no. 3 (1926): 113.

14. *School Lunch and Milk Programs: Hearings before a Subcommittee
    of the Committee on Agriculture and Forestry, United States Senate, 78th
    Congress, 2nd Session, on S. 1820 and S. 1824* (1944), 7.

15. See, for example, David R. Just and Brian Wansink, "Smarter Lunch-
    rooms: Using Behavioral Economics to Improve Meal Selection," *Choices*
    24, no. 3 (2009), available at http://www.choicesmagazine.org/magazine
    /article.php?article=87.

16. A key challenge in reconstructing the histories of school meal programs
    prior to federal involvement is that there are very few detailed records.
    What records survive tend to be fragmented across archival sources, offi-
    cial reports, journal publications, and newspaper or magazine articles, often
    with significant gaps in coverage. Moreover, there was no systematic docu-
    mentation of the views of teachers, parents, or students in most locations.
    Thus, while exhaustive research has made it possible to understand how
    and why school meal programs were implemented in a few locations, it
    is far more difficult—and in most cases impossible—to say anything with
    certainty about the effects of school feeding on child hunger or malnutri-
    tion, about the effects of student race on access to school meals, or about the
    extent to which the small number of school meal programs for which there
    is documentation were representative of such programs nationally.

Chapter 1 — "The Old-Fashioned Lunch Box . . . Seems Likely to Be Extinct"

1. Horace P. Makechnie, "Problems in Feeding School Children," *Journal of the American Medical Association* 30, no. 2 (8 January 1898): 56.

2. On the history of school hygiene in this period, see Richard A.
   Meckel, *Classrooms and Clinics: Urban Schools and the Protection and
   Promotion of Child Health, 1870–1930* (New Brunswick, NJ: Rutgers Uni-
   versity Press, 2013).

3. Jessie P. Rich, *The Problem of the School Luncheon, Pt. I,* Bulletin
   338, Extension Series 48 (Austin: University of Texas, 1914), 3.

4. Recent studies have generally supported this claim. See, for example, A. F. Meyers et al., "School Breakfast Program and School Performance," *American Journal of the Diseases of Children* 143, no. 10 (1989): 1234–1239; S. Anzman-Frasca et al., "Estimating Impacts of a Breakfast in the Classroom Program on School Outcomes," *JAMA Pediatrics* 169, no. 1 (2015): 71–77.

5. Meckel, *Classrooms and Clinics*; William J. Reese, *Power and the Promise of School Reform: Grassroots Movements during the Progressive Era* (Boston: Routledge & Kegan Paul, 1986).

6. Meckel, *Classrooms and Clinics*; Louise Stevens Bryant, *School Feeding: Its History and Practice at Home and Abroad* (Philadelphia: J. B. Lippincott, 1913); Bernard Harris, *The Health of the Schoolchild: A History of the School Medical Service in England and Wales* (Buckingham: Open University Press, 1995); Hideharu Umehara, *Gesunde Schule und Gesunde Kinder: Schulhygiene in Düsseldorf, 1880–1933* (Essen: Klartext Verlag, 2013).

7. In France and Germany, concern about declining birth rates also contributed to the development of child health and welfare programs.

8. See, for example, Tracy L. Steffes, *School, Society, and State: A New Education to Govern Modern America, 1890–1940* (Chicago: University of Chicago Press, 2012).

9. *What American Cities Are Doing for the Health of School Children, Part I: Medical Inspection* (New York: Russell Sage Foundation, Division of Child Hygiene, 1912), 5.

10. Robert W. Hastings, "Medical Inspection of Schools," *American Journal of Public Health* 2, no. 12 (1912): 973; A. R. Ruis, "'Children with Half-Starved Bodies' and the Assessment of Malnutrition in the United States, 1890–1950," *Bulletin of the History of Medicine* 87, no. 3 (2013): 380–408.

11. Meckel, *Classrooms and Clinics*, 101.

12. Anna Barrows, "The Lunch-Room in the High School," *School Review* 13, no. 3 (1905): 213.

13. Avery M. Guest and Stuart E. Tolnay, "Children's Roles and Fertility: Late Nineteenth-Century United States," *Social Science History* 7 (1983): 355–380.

14. Viviana A. Zelizer, *Pricing the Priceless Child: The Changing Social Value of Children* (New York: Basic Books, 1985), 23.

15. Ernest Bryant Hoag and Lewis M. Terman, *Health Work in the Schools* (Boston: Houghton Mifflin, 1914), 120.

16. Reese, *Power and the Promise of School Reform*, 212 ff.

17. S. Josephine Baker, "The Relation of the War to the Nourishment of Children," *New York Medical Journal* 107, no. 7 (1918): 289.

18. *The School Lunch* (Columbus: Ohio State University, Agricultural Extension Service, 1922), 3. Note that in this context, "retardation" referred only to slow progress, not necessarily to a cognitive impairment or disability.

19. Mary Swartz Rose, *Feeding the Family* (New York: Macmillan, 1916), 154.

20. Edward Beecher Hooker, "The Malnutrition of School Children and Its Physical and Social Consequences," *Clinique* 27, no. 10 (1906): 586.

21. Ira S. Wile, "School Lunches," *Journal of Home Economics* 2, no. 2 (1910): 167.

22. On the history of eugenics in the United States, see Daniel J. Kevles, *In the Name of Eugenics: Genetics and the Uses of Human Heredity* (New York: Alfred A. Knopf, 1985); Edward J. Larson, *Sex, Race, and Science: Eugenics in the Deep South* (Baltimore: Johns Hopkins University Press, 1995); Alexandra Minna Stern, *Eugenic Nation: Faults and Frontiers of Better Breeding in Modern America* (Berkeley: University of California Press, 2005).

23. "How the Plan of Providing Lunch for New York School Children Has Worked," *Washington Post Magazine*, 3 July 1910, 1.

24. Ellen H. Richards, *Euthenics, the Science of Controllable Environment: A Plea for Better Living Conditions as a First Step toward Higher Human Efficiency* (Boston: Whitcomb & Barrows, 1910).

25. Hoag and Terman, *Health Work in the Schools*, 4.

26. This linkage between the individual body and the body politic was global in scope, becoming a central element of identity formation not only in the imperial nations of Europe, Japan, and the United States but also in countries like China and India, which were beginning to develop national identities. See, for example, Harvey Green, *Fit for America: Health, Fitness, Sport, and American Society* (New York: Pantheon Books, 1986); Andrew D. Morris, *Marrow of the Nation: A History of Sport and Physical Culture in Republican China* (Berkeley: University of California Press, 2004); Claire E. Nolte, *The Sokol in the Czech Lands to 1914: Training for the Nation* (New York: Palgrave Macmillan, 2002); Tricia Starks, *The Body Soviet: Propaganda, Hygiene, and the Revolutionary State* (Madison: University of Wisconsin Press, 2008).

27. Lucy H. Gillett, *Diet for the School Child* (Washington, DC: U.S. Bureau of Education, 1919), 1.

28. Barrows, "The Lunch-Room in the High School," 213.

29. "New York Labor Organizations Back Comprehensive Program of Education," *School Life* 1, no. 6 (1918): 3.

30. Ira S. Wile, "The Relative Physical Advantages of School Lunches in Elementary and Secondary Schools," *Bulletin of the American Academy of Medicine* 14 (1913): 149.

31. Rich, *Problem of the School Luncheon*, 6. See also Alice C. Boughton, *Household Arts and School Lunches* (Cleveland, OH: Cleveland Foundation, 1916), 165.

32. Wile, "School Lunches and Medical Inspection," 345.

33. Lewis W. Rapeer, *Educational Hygiene from the Pre-School Period to the University* (New York: Charles Scribner's Sons, 1915), 280.

34. Judith Walzer Leavitt, *The Healthiest City: Milwaukee and the Politics of Health Reform* (Princeton: Princeton University Press, 1982), 190 ff.
35. Mrs. Frederic Schoff, "School Luncheons," *National Congress of Mothers Magazine* 3, no. 3 (1908): 81.
36. "Hot Lunches for School Children," *Spirit Lake (IA) Beacon*, 1 February 1917, 1.
37. See, for example, Josephine Grenier, "School Luncheons," *Harper's Bazaar* 37 (1903): 979–981; Ida C. Allen, "The Children's School Luncheons," *Ladies' Home Journal* 23 (1916): 83; Caroline L. Hunt and Mabel Ward, *School Lunches* (Washington, DC: U.S. Department of Agriculture, 1916); Lucy H. Gillett, *Diet for the School Child* (Washington, DC: U.S. Bureau of Education, 1919).
38. Josephine Grenier, "Children's School Luncheons," *Harper's Bazaar* 40 (1906): 951.
39. "Cheap Meals at the Normal," *Los Angeles Times* (21 May 1905), 16.
40. "Serving Hot Lunches in Schools Started in Europe and Is Now Spreading in the U.S.," *Fresno Morning Republican* (26 October 1913), 16.
41. "Problem of the Schoolboy's Lunch Basket," *New York Times* (12 January 1913), X13.
42. Mary Swartz Rose, *Feeding the Family* (New York: Macmillan, 1916), 155.
43. Albertina Bechmann, "The First Penny Lunch," *Journal of Home Economics* 25, no. 9 (1933): 762.
44. Lydia J. Roberts, *The Child Health School Conducted in the School of Education of the University of Chicago during the Summer of 1920* (Washington, DC: U.S. Bureau of Education, 1923), 23.
45. George T. Palmer, "Detroit's Experience with Undernourished School Children," *American Journal of Public Health* 11 (1921): 135.
46. Boughton, *Household Arts and School Lunches*, 116–117.
47. Frank R. Keefer, "Causes of Army Rejections: What Health Officers Can Do to Remedy Conditions," *American Journal of Public Health* 10, no. 3 (1920): 236–239. See also *Defects Found in Drafted Men* (Washington, DC: U.S. Government Printing Office, 1919); Frederick L. Hoffman, *Army Anthropometry and Medical Rejection Statistics* (Washington, DC: National Research Council, 1918).
48. Rupert Blue, "Are We Physically Fit? United States Handicapped in Coming Period of Commercial and Industrial Competition," *American Journal of Public Health* 9, no. 9 (1919): 642; Taliaferro Clark, "The Need and Opportunity for Physical Education in Rural Communities," *American Physical Education Review* 24, no. 9 (1919): 440. Similar conclusions were drawn by British authorities. See, for example, J. M. Hamill, *Diet in Relation to Normal Nutrition* (London: Ministry of Health, 1921), 3.
49. Alice H. Wood, "Nutrition Classes in the Chicago Schools," *Modern Medicine* 2, no. 5 (1920): 388.

50. Rama V. Bennett, "An Analysis of the Development of the Interest in Malnutrition of Children as Reflected in Periodical Literature" (thesis, University of Chicago, 1925), data in appendix.

51. Frank C. Doig, "School Cafeterias in Seattle," *American City* 22, no. 2 (1920): 123.

52. "Hot Lunch Helps Young America Get His Lessons: Five Cents Buys a Meal at City Schools," *Chicago Daily Tribune*, 17 October 1930, 24.

53. "Cold Lunch Passing," *Sandusky (OH) Star-Journal* (21 August 1919), 11. See also Reinette Lovewell, "Substitute for the Dinner Pail," *Technical World Magazine*, September 1914, 52.

54. Helen Hollister, "Training Women to Manage Lunch Rooms," *New York Times*, 9 February 1913, X10.

55. Edwin L. Miller, "The Lunch-Room at the Englewood High School," *School Review* 13, no. 3 (1905): 202.

56. "High School Lunch: Ice Cream and Tamales Not Filling the Bill," *Los Angeles Times*, 23 March 1901, A3.

57. "Solves Lunch Issue: Plan for Knocking Out High School Pickle Trade," *Decatur (IA) Daily Review* (12 January 1900), 2.

58. "High School Lunch Room: Pupils to Be Hygienically Fed at Low Prices," *New Haven (CT) Evening Register*, 8 November 1897, 1.

59. Gladys Stillman, *Milk Drinking Survey of Rural School Children* (Madison: Wisconsin State Department of Public Health, Nutrition Division, 1934), Nutrition Division Files, Series 2712, Box 2, Folder 34, Archives of the Wisconsin State Historical Society.

60. Elizabeth Farrell, "School Luncheons in the Special Classes of the Public Schools," *Charities* 13, no. 24 (1905): 569–570.

61. "Feeding a Hungry High School," *San Antonio Light*, 23 January 1916, 20.

62. Alice C. Boughton, "The Administration of School Lunches in Cities," Fourth International Congress on School Hygiene, Buffalo, NY, 1913, *Transactions*, vol. 5 (Buffalo: Courier, 1914), 307. The figure given is in unadjusted dollars.

63. "Millions of Dollars Invested in the Street Corner Business," *New Orleans Daily Picayune*, 7 June 1903, 23. Figures given are in unadjusted dollars. Approximately one-quarter of the street stands were located in New York City.

64. "Dinner Pail No More: Laborer Buys His Lunch of Pushcart Man," *Cleveland Plain Dealer*, 27 December 1903, 15.

65. *Women in the Candy Industry in Chicago and St. Louis* (Washington, DC: U.S. Department of Labor, 1923), 1.

66. Philip J. Hilts, *Protecting America's Health: The FDA, Business, and One Hundred Years of Regulation* (New York: Alfred A. Knopf, 2003), 22–23. On the history of food analysis and health reform, see also Oscar E. Anderson Jr., *The Health of a Nation: Harvey W. Wiley and the Fight for Pure Food* (Chicago: University of Chicago Press, 1958); Lorine Swainston

Goodwin, *The Pure Food, Drink, and Drug Crusaders, 1879–1914* (Jefferson, NC: McFarland, 1999); Mitchell Okun, *Fair Play in the Marketplace: The First Battle for Pure Food and Drugs* (Dekalb: Northern Illinois University Press, 1986).

67. Jessie P. Rich, *The Problem of the School Luncheon, Pt. II*, Bulletin 339, Extension Series 49 (Austin: University of Texas, 1914), 3.

68. *Report and Handbook of the Department of Health of the City of Chicago for the Years 1911 to 1918 Inclusive* (1919), 979–980. In 1917, the city of Chicago prohibited saloons from offering free lunches.

Chapter 2 — (II)Legal Lunches

1. Board of Education of the City of Chicago, *Reports on Underfed Children* (1908), 5, 14–15.

2. "Ghetto" was not a generic term in this case but referred to a specific neighborhood on the Near West Side, so I have retained the capitalization to avoid confusion.

3. "The Hunger Problem in the Public Schools: What a Canvass of Six Big Cities Reveals," *North American Magazine*, 21 May 1905.

4. *Report of the Department of Health of the City of Chicago for the Years 1907, 1908, 1909, 1910*, 144 ff., 167–168.

5. Board of Education of the City of Chicago, *Reports on Underfed Children*, 7–10. See also "Hungry School Children in Chicago," *Charities and the Commons* 20 (1908): 93–96.

6. "Five Moves Made to Allay Hunger," *Chicago Daily Tribune*, 8 October 1908, 7.

7. Andrew Carnegie, *The Gospel of Wealth and Other Timely Essays* (New York: Century, 1901), 15.

8. On the history of aid societies and organized charity in this period, see Brent Ruswick, *Almost Worthy: The Poor, Paupers, and the Science of Charity in America, 1877–1917* (Bloomington: Indiana University Press, 2012); Lawrence J. Friedman and Mark D. McGarvie, eds., *Charity, Philanthropy, and Civility in American History* (Cambridge: Cambridge University Press, 2003); Kathleen D. McCarthy, *Noblesse Oblige: Charity and Cultural Philanthropy in Chicago, 1849–1929* (Chicago: University of Chicago Press, 1982); Kenneth L. Kusmer, "The Functions of Organized Charity in the Progressive Era: Chicago as a Case Study," *Journal of American History* 60, no. 3 (1973): 657–678.

9. Judith Walzer Leavitt, *The Healthiest City: Milwaukee and the Politics of Health Reform* (Princeton: Princeton University Press, 1982), 190 ff., 205.

10. "Five Moves Made to Allay Hunger."

11. Edwin L. Miller, "The Lunch-Room at the Englewood High School," *School Review* 13, no. 3 (1905): 206.

12. Board of Education of the City of Chicago, *Reports on Underfed Children*, 3.

13. *Printed Record of the Board of Education of the City of St. Louis*, 12 January 1904, 286.

14. The CSEC was originally called the Permanent School Extension Committee.

15. *Report of the Chicago Permanent School Extension Committee, 1911*, 10.

16. Mary J. Herrick, *The Chicago Schools: A Social and Political History* (Beverly Hills, CA: Sage, 1971), 114.

17. George S. Counts, *School and Society in Chicago* (New York: Harcourt Brace Jovanovich, 1928), 66.

18. *Proceedings of the Board of Education of the City of Chicago*, 1 November 1911, 278; *Report of the Chicago Permanent School Extension Committee, 1911*, 10–11.

19. Gordan Seagrove, "Chicago and Its City of Mysterious Death," *Chicago Daily Tribune*, 3 October 1915, D1.

20. Mary Katherine Synon, "Children of Little Italy," *Chicago Daily Tribune*, 30 August 1903, 43.

21. Ibid.

22. James R. Grossman, Ann Durkin Keating, and Janice L. Reiff, eds., *The Encyclopedia of Chicago* (Chicago: University of Chicago Press, 2004), 675–676; Helen Rankin Jeter, "Tenement Rents," in *The Tenements of Chicago, 1908–1935*, ed. Edith Abbott (Chicago: University of Chicago Press, 1936), 276–277; Robert G. Spinney, *City of Big Shoulders: A History of Chicago* (Dekalb: Northern Illinois University Press, 2000), 130–133.

23. "Many Seek Penny Lunches," *Chicago Daily Tribune*, 16 December 1910, 7.

24. *Report of the Chicago School Extension Committee, 1913*, 5.

25. Ibid.

26. *Report of the Chicago School Extension Committee, 1912*, 4.

27. Louise Stevens Bryant, *School Feeding: Its History and Practice at Home and Abroad* (Philadelphia: J. B. Lippincott, 1913), 233 ff.

28. *Report of the Chicago School Extension Committee, 1912*, 4.

29. *Report of the Chicago School Extension Committee, 1914*, 3.

30. *Proceedings of the Board of Education of the City of Chicago*, 20 November 1907, 307.

31. "Report of the Sub-Committee on Penny Lunches," *Proceedings of the Board of Education of the City of Chicago*, 5 November 1914, 443.

32. "Penny School Lunch Puts Out H.C.L. in a Round," *Chicago Daily Tribune*, 3 October 1917, 13; *Proceedings of the Board of Education of the City of Chicago*, 15 September 1915, 833.

33. "Penny School Lunch Puts Out H.C.L. in a Round."

34. *Proceedings of the Board of Education of the City of Chicago*, 23 November 1917, 668.

35. *Laws of the State of Illinois* (Springfield, 1893), 180.

36. A similar case, with the same ruling, was heard before the Mississippi Supreme Court: *Thompson v. Lamar County Agricultural High School,* 117 Miss. 621, 78 So. 547 (1918).

37. *Proceedings of the Board of Education of the City of Chicago,* 23 November 1917, 668–672.

38. *Proceedings of the Board of Education of the City of Chicago,* 26 November 1917, 766.

39. Those states were California, Colorado, Connecticut, Indiana, Massachusetts, Michigan, Missouri, New Jersey, New York, North Carolina, Ohio, Pennsylvania, Rhode Island, Vermont, Washington, and Wisconsin.

40. "Governor Disapproves School Lunch Bill," *Grand Rapids Tribune,* 6 October 1919, 4.

41. C. P. Cary, *School Law Supplement Giving the Amendments and New School Laws as Enacted by the Legislature of 1917* (Madison, WI: Democrat Printing, 1917), ch. 427 § 486t.

42. A third state, Massachusetts, assigned this power to local governments beginning in 1915: "The city council of a city and the selectmen of a town may provide meals or lunches free or at no more than cost price to children attending public schools, and cities and towns may appropriate money for this purpose. This act shall be submitted to the voters of any city or town at a municipal election in any year if a petition to that effect, signed by not less than 5 per cent of voters, is filed with the city or town clerk." See William R. Hood, Stephen B. Weeks, and A. Sidney Ford, *Digest of Laws Relating to Public Education in Force January 1, 1915* (Washington, DC: U.S. Department of the Interior, Bureau of Education, 1916), 594.

43. *Proceedings of the Board of Education of the City of Chicago,* 23 November 1917, 663–664.

44. *Proceedings of the Board of Education of the City of Chicago,* 12 March 1919, 275.

45. *Proceedings of the Board of Education of the City of Chicago,* 12 July 1921, 15.

46. *Proceedings of the Board of Education of the City of Chicago,* 25 March 1925, 950–951.

47. W. A. Evans, "How to Keep Well: The School Lunch," *Chicago Daily Tribune,* 30 May 1926, 6.

48. "No State shall make or enforce any law which shall abridge the privileges or immunities of citizens of the United States; nor shall any State deprive any person of life, liberty, or property, without due process of law; nor deny to any person within its jurisdiction the equal protection of the laws."

49. *Goodman v. School District No. 1, City and County of Denver, et al.,* 32 F.2d 586 (1929). See also *Speyer et al. v. School District No. 1, City and County of Denver,* 82 Colo. 534 (1927).

50. *Ralph v. Orleans Parish School Board,* 104 So. 491 (1925).

51. *Krueger v. Board of Education of the City of St. Louis,* 274 So. 811 (1925).

52. *Special Acts of the Houston Board of Education* (1923), ch. 91, § 1, Rev. Stat. 1925, art. 2780, as cited in *Bishop v. Houston Independent School District,* 29 S.W.2d 312, 314 (1930).

53. *Bozeman et al. v. Morrow et al.,* 30 S.W.2d 657 (1931).

54. *Hallett et al. v. Post Printing and Publishing Co.,* 12 A.L.R. 919 (1920).

55. Ernest Bryant Hoag and Lewis M. Terman, *Health Work in the Schools* (Cambridge, MA: Riverside Press, 1914); Lawrence A. Averill, "The School Clinic," *American Journal of School Hygiene* 1 (1917): 93–99.

56. Stephen Woolworth, "A Radical Proposition: The Brief but Exceptional History of the Seattle School Clinic, 1914–21," *Journal of the History of Medicine and Allied Sciences* 68, no. 2 (2013): 227–265.

57. *McGilvra et al. v. Seattle School District No. 1,* 12 A.L.R. 913 (1921).

58. American Child Health Association, *Report of the Chicago Health Education Conference, 1925* (New York: ACHA, 1926), 261.

59. "Hot Lunch Helps Young America Get His Lessons: Five Cents Buys a Meal at City Schools," *Chicago Daily Tribune,* 17 October 1930, 24.

60. *Annual Report of the Board of Education of the City of St. Louis, Missouri, 1925–26,* 504, 507.

61. Bryant, *School Feeding,* 173–174.

62. *Annual Report of the Board of Education of the City of St. Louis, Missouri, 1925–26,* 503.

63. Ibid., 510–11.

64. *Annual Report of the Superintendent of Schools of the City of Chicago, 1923–24,* 45.

65. *Proceedings of the Board of Education of the City of Chicago,* 26 December 1934, 446; 14 May 1941, 1547.

66. *Proceedings of the Board of Education of the City of Chicago,* 14 May 1941, 1544.

67. Leone Pazourek, "A Plan for Improving School Lunches," *Nutrition News* 4, no. 1 (1940): 3.

68. This is similar to the way many states maintain bridges for automobile traffic: initial construction costs come from tax revenues, but most subsequent costs are subsidized by usage taxes, e.g., tolls.

Chapter 3 — Menus for the Melting Pot

1. Lillian D. Wald, "The Feeding of School Children," *Charities and the Commons* 20 (1908): 371.

2. Michael J. Eula, "Failure of American Food Reformers among Italian Immigrants in New York City, 1891–1897," *Italian Americana* 18, no. 1 (2000): 86–99. See also Harvey Levenstein, *Revolution at the Table: The Transformation of the American Diet* (New York: Oxford University Press, 1988), ch. 4.

3. With the exception of Chicago, few cities had a coordinated school lunch program as extensive as New York's prior to federal intervention.

4. Leonard P. Ayres, *The Cleveland School Survey: Summary Volume* (Cleveland, OH: Cleveland Foundation, 1917), 234.

5. For a recent discussion of the ambiguity between public and private in responsibility for municipal services, see Jessica Wang, "Dogs and the Making of the American State: Voluntary Association, State Power, and the Politics of Animal Control in New York City, 1850–1920," *Journal of American History* 98, no. 4 (2012): 998–1024.

6. See, for example, Suellen M. Hoy, *Chasing Dirt: The American Pursuit of Cleanliness* (New York: Oxford University Press, 1995); Nancy J. Tomes, *The Gospel of Germs: Men, Women, and the Microbe in American Life* (Cambridge: Harvard University Press, 1998).

7. Jane Jacobs, *The Death and Life of Great American Cities* (New York: Random House, 1961). On the expansion of public health police powers, see, for example, Philip J. Hilts, *Protecting America's Health: The FDA, Business, and One Hundred Years of Regulation* (New York: Alfred A. Knopf, 2003); Judith Walzer Leavitt, *Typhoid Mary: Captive to the Public's Health* (Boston: Beacon Press, 1996); Nayan Shah, *Contagious Divides: Epidemics and Race in San Francisco's Chinatown* (Berkeley: University of California Press, 2001).

8. On the history of "baby saving" campaigns and scientific motherhood, see Rima D. Apple, *Perfect Motherhood: Science and Childrearing in America* (New Brunswick, NJ: Rutgers University Press, 2006); Molly Ladd-Taylor, *Mother-Work: Women, Child Welfare, and the State, 1890–1930* (Urbana: University of Illinois Press, 1994); Richard A. Meckel, *Save the Babies: American Public Health Reform and the Prevention of Infant Mortality, 1850–1929* (Baltimore: Johns Hopkins University Press, 1990); Jacqueline H. Wolf, *Don't Kill Your Baby: Public Health and the Decline of Breastfeeding in the Nineteenth and Twentieth Centuries* (Columbus: Ohio State University Press, 2001).

9. Tracy L. Steffes, *School, Society, and State: A New Education to Govern Modern America, 1890–1940* (Chicago: University of Chicago Press, 2012), 3. For a discussion of these issues in the context of medicine and public health, see Stephen Woolworth, "A Radical Proposition: The Brief but Exceptional History of the Seattle School Clinic, 1914–21," *Journal of the History of Medicine and Allied Sciences* 68, no. 2 (2013): 227–265.

10. Diane Ravitch, *The Great School Wars: A History of the New York City Public Schools* (New York: Basic Books, 1974), 183, 189–190.

11. Edward T. Devine, "The Underfed Child in the Schools," *Charities and the Commons* 20 (1908): 413. See also Leonard P. Ayres, *The Relation of Physical Defects to School Progress* (New York: Russell Sage Foundation, Division of Education, 1909), 8.

12. *Annual Report of the Board of Health for the City of New York, 1909–1912* (each year published separately); E. Mather Sill, "Malnutrition in

School Children in New York City," *Journal of Home Economics* 1, no. 4 (1909): 370.

13. "Say School Children Are Not Starving," *New York Times*, 11 June 1908, 4.

14. For a discussion of the emergence of malnutrition as a public health problem, see Jeffrey P. Brosco, "Weight Charts and Well Child Care: When the Pediatrician Became the Expert in Child Health," in *Formative Years: Children's Health in the United States, 1880–2000*, ed. Alexandra Minna Stern and Howard Markel (Ann Arbor: University of Michigan Press, 2004), 91–120; Richard A. Meckel, "Politics, Policy, and the Measuring of Child Health: Child Malnutrition in the Great Depression," in *Healing the World's Children: Interdisciplinary Perspectives on Child Health in the Twentieth Century*, ed. Janet Golden, Cynthia R. Comacchio, and George Weisz (Montreal: McGill-Queen's University Press, 2008), 235–252; A. R. Ruis, "'Children with Half-Starved Bodies' and the Assessment of Malnutrition in the United States, 1890–1950," *Bulletin of the History of Medicine* 87, no. 3 (2013): 380–408.

15. Mabel Hyde Kittredge, "School Lunch Problem, Solved, Now Strikes a Snag," *New York Times*, 12 January 1913, SM6.

16. Barbara L. Ciccarelli, "Mabel Hyde Kittredge," in *American National Biography*, ed. John A. Garraty and Mark C. Carnes (New York: Oxford University Press, 1999), 12:782–783.

17. Three cents was inexpensive, but even that would have been a lot for some of the city's poorest children. A room in a tenement house, the cheapest form of housing, cost between three and six dollars per week in rent, and an unskilled laborer could expect to make around seven dollars per week.

18. Mabel Hyde Kittredge, "Experiments with School Lunches in New York City," *Journal of Home Economics* 2, no. 2 (1910): 174–175.

19. Jeff Kisseloff, *You Must Remember This: An Oral History of Manhattan from the 1890s to World War II* (San Diego: Harcourt Brace Jovanovich, 1989), 563–564. See also Katharine Anthony, *Mothers Who Must Earn* (New York: Russell Sage Foundation, 1914), 9–10, 145.

20. Olivia Howard Dunbar, "Three-Cent Luncheons for School-Children," *Outlook* 97 (1911): 34–35; Kittredge, "Experiments with School Lunches," 177.

21. Edward F. Brown, *The School Lunch Service in New York City* (New York: New York City Department of Education, Division of Reference and Research, 1914), 6.

22. Kittredge, "Experiments with School Lunches," 176. "Postu" is likely a misspelling of "postum," a toasted grain beverage marketed as an alternative to coffee. It is most likely not a misspelling of "pasta," as Kittredge does not use the term elsewhere.

23. Kenneth T. Jackson and Stanley K. Schultz, eds., *Cities in American History* (New York: Alfred A. Knopf, 1972), 180.

24. Jacob Riis, *How the Other Half Lives: Studies among the Tenements of New York City* (New York: Charles Scribner's Sons, 1890), 15.

25. Emma Winslow, as quoted in Viviana A. Zelizer, *The Social Meaning of Money* (Princeton: Princeton University Press, 1997), 122.

26. Harry Golden, *Ess, Ess, Mein Kindt* (New York: G. P. Putnam's Sons, 1963), 86.

27. Kittredge, "Experiments with School Lunches," 176.

28. *Annual Report of the [New York] City Superintendent of Schools, 1912*, 186.

29. Louise Stevens Bryant, *School Feeding: Its History and Practice at Home and Abroad* (Philadelphia: J. B. Lippincott, 1913), 150; Dunbar, "Three-Cent Luncheons," 36.

30. Kittredge, "Experiments with School Lunches," 176–177.

31. *Annual Report of the [New York] City Superintendent of Schools, 1912*, 180.

32. Ruth S. True, *Boyhood and Lawlessness* (New York: Russell Sage Foundation, 1914), 75.

33. Bryant, *School Feeding*, 248.

34. True, *Boyhood and Lawlessness*, 75.

35. Kittredge, "School Lunch Problem." See also Donald B. Armstrong, "The Hygienic Features of School Lunches," *New York Medical Journal*, 18 September 1915: 604.

36. "Two-Cent Luncheon Delights Roosevelt," *New York Times*, 16 April 1913, 1.

37. Kittredge, "School Lunch Problem"; Kittredge, "Experiments with School Lunches," 177.

38. Mabel Hyde Kittredge, "Relation of Menus to Standard Dietaries," Fourth International Congress on School Hygiene, Buffalo, NY, 1913, *Transactions*, vol. 5 (Buffalo: Courier, 1914), 313.

39. Ira S. Wile, "The Relative Physical Advantages of School Lunches in Elementary and Secondary Schools," *Bulletin of the American Academy of Medicine* 14 (1913): 154.

40. Kittredge, "Relation of Menus to Standard Dietaries," 313.

41. Kittredge, "School Lunch Problem."

42. Letter from Margaret Anne Poole to Mrs. Ingram, 27 November 1912, Community Service Society Archives, MS 0273, Box 49, Folder 325.2, Columbia University Rare Book and Manuscript Collection, New York. See also *Shall the Schools Serve Lunches?* (New York: New York City Public Education Association, 1913), 1.

43. Superintendent was the highest administrative position in the Education Department, but the superintendent's role was to manage personnel and enforce (not establish) policy. Only the Board of Education, city hall, or the state legislature could effect permanent change in school policy.

44. *Annual Report of the [New York] City Superintendent of Schools, 1912*, 186–189.

45. See chapter 2 for a discussion of the legal status of publicly funded school meal programs.

46. On the history of the AICP, see Dorothy G. Becker, "The Visitor to the New York City Poor, 1843–1920: The Role and Contributions of Volunteer Visitors of the New York Association for the Improvement of the Condition of the Poor, State Charities Aid Association, and New York Charity Organization Society" (D.S.W. thesis, Columbia University, 1960); Lilian Brandt, *Growth and Development of AICP and COS* (New York: Community Service Society, 1942); John Duffy, *A History of Public Health in New York City, 1866–1966* (New York: Russell Sage Foundation, 1974), ch. 17.

47. Brown, "School Lunch Service in New York City," 13.

48. *Annual Report of the [New York] City Superintendent of Schools, 1912*, 187.

49. "Lunches for School-Children," *Outlook* 112 (1916): 361.

50. Letter from Haven Emerson to Mabel Hyde Kittredge, 4 June 1917, Community Service Society Archives, MS 0273, Box 49, Folder 325.2, Columbia University Rare Book and Manuscript Collection, New York.

51. On the transition of control of school health services from boards of health to boards of education, see Luther Halsey Gulick and Leonard P. Ayres, *Medical Inspection of Schools* (New York: Russell Sage Foundation, 1908), 142 ff.

52. Brown, "School Lunch Service in New York City," 9.

53. *Annual Report of the [New York] Association for Improving the Condition of the Poor, 1914*, 106.

54. "Two-Cent Luncheon Delights Roosevelt," 1.

55. *Annual Report of the [New York] City Superintendent of Schools, 1914*, 174–176.

56. *Journal of the Board of Education of the City of New York*, 1 February 1915, 233; 14 April 1915, 649.

57. *Journal of the Board of Education of the City of New York*, 11 August 1915, 1396–1398.

58. S. Josephine Baker, "The Relation of the War to the Nourishment of Children," *New York Medical Journal*, 16 February 1918, 291.

59. *Annual Report of the Board of Health of the City of New York, 1918*, 126–128; "Underfed Children Problem in Schools," *New York Times*, 23 December 1917, 18. On the changes in diagnostics and surveillance of malnutrition, see Ruis, "'Children with Half-Starved Bodies,'" 388–389.

60. S. Josephine Baker, *Fighting for Life* (New York: Macmillan, 1939), 170.

61. *Annual Report of the Board of Health of the City of New York, 1918*, 159–161; "School Luncheons before Aldermen," *New York Times*, 15 February 1918, 9; "May Favor School Lunch," *New York Times*, 26 March 1918, 6; "Plea for School Lunches," *New York Times*, 9 August 1918, 6; "Nation's Duty to Preserve the Health of Children," *New York Times*, 11 August 1918, 31.

62. *Annual Report of the [New York] Association for Improving the Condition of the Poor, 1919*, 22.

63. Alice C. Boughton, *Suggested Program and Recommendations for an Experiment in School Feeding to Be Conducted by the Board of Education of the City of New York* (New York: Child Health Organization, 1919), Community Service Society Archives, MS 0273, Box 50, Folder 325.2, Columbia University Rare Book and Manuscript Collection, New York. As early as 1913, the SLC had presented the board with a plan for directing school foodservice in the public schools. See *Shall the Schools Serve Lunches?*, 5.

64. Letter from Bailey B. Burritt to Albert G. Milbank, 21 March 1919, Community Service Society Archives, MS 0273, Box 49, Folder 325.2, Columbia University Rare Book and Manuscript Collection, New York.

65. Ibid.

66. "'Penny Lunches' in Schools Halted by a Technicality," *New York Evening World*, 5 December 1919, 27.

67. John C. Gebhart, *Malnutrition and School Feeding* (Washington, DC: U.S. Department of the Interior, Bureau of Education, 1921), 14–18; E. H. Lewinski-Corwin and Elizabeth V. Cunningham, *Thirty Years in Community Service, 1911–1941* (New York: New York Academy of Medicine, 1942), 89; Diane Ravitch, *The Great School Wars: A History of the New York City Public Schools* (New York: Basic Books, 1974), 195–196, 228–230.

68. *Annual Report of the [New York] City Superintendent of Schools, 1926*, 188–189.

69. Gebhart, *Malnutrition and School Feeding*, 13–14. For more such menus, see Rowena Wellman, "Feeding Ten Thousand Underweight Children," *American Food Journal* 20, no. 2 (1925): 77.

70. James P. Hornaday, "School Lunch Is Important," *Bedford (PA) Gazette*, 1 October 1920, 3.

71. *Health for School Children: Report of Advisory Committee on Health Education* (Washington, DC: National Child Health Council, 1923), 30.

72. Mary G. McCormick, *The Rural Hot Lunch and the Nutrition of the Rural Child* (Albany: State University of New York, 1919), 2.

73. On the history of immigrant foodways, see Hasia R. Diner, *Hungering for America: Italian, Irish, and Jewish Foodways in the Age of Migration* (Cambridge: Harvard University Press, 2001); Donna R. Gabaccia, *We Are What We Eat: Ethnic Food and the Making of Americans* (Cambridge: Harvard University Press, 1998).

74. Leonard Covello and Guido D'Agostino, *The Heart Is the Teacher* (New York: McGraw-Hill, 1958), 24–25.

75. John Fante, "The Odyssey of a Wop," *American Mercury* 30, no. 12 (1933): 91. Covello, too, had conflicting attitudes about Italian food; like Fante, he recalled being "always ashamed of the bulky sandwiches of crusty Italian bread heaped with salami, cheese or Italian sausage. We used to keep them hidden or eat them even before we got to school, so that our friends of the white-bread-and-ham upbringing would not laugh at us" (Covello and D'Agostino, *The Heart Is the Teacher*, 70.)

76. Anzia Yezierska, *Bread Givers: A Struggle between a Father of the Old World and a Daughter of the New* (New York: Persea Books, 1925), 165–167, 173. See also Deborah Israel, "Food, Hunger, and Identity in Jewish Women Immigrants' Autobiography," in *You Are What You Eat: Literary Probes into the Palate*, ed. Annette M. Magid (Newcastle, Eng.: Cambridge Scholars, 2008), 238–258.

77. Al Hirshberg and Sammy Aaronson, *As High as My Heart: The Sammy Aaronson Story* (New York: Coward-McCann, 1957), 18–19.

78. The SLC had a separate subcommittee for Brooklyn and Queens, which was operating approximately twenty lunch programs as late as 1917, but virtually no records of its activities seem to have survived. See *Annual Report of the American Association for Improving the Condition of the Poor* (New York, 1915), 85; Gebhart, *Malnutrition and School Feeding*, 17.

79. *Annual Report of the [New York] City Superintendent of Schools, 1925*, 281.

80. "School Lunch Protest," *New York Times*, 23 March 1927, 24; *Annual Report of the New York Academy of Medicine, 1926*, 173.

81. "School Lunches Are Called Unfit," *New York Times*, 31 October 1927, 21.

82. *Annual Report of the [New York] City Superintendent of Schools, 1927*, 351; "Moves to Reform School Lunch Plan: Situation Called Acute," *New York Times*, 23 November 1927, 7.

83. *Annual Report of the [New York] City Superintendent of Schools, 1929*, 213–214.

84. Interestingly, New York City recently reinvented this approach to school lunches. See Kim Severson, "Schools' Toughest Test: Cooking," *New York Times*, 30 September 2009, D1.

Chapter 4 — Food for the Farm Belt

1. Harper Lee, *To Kill a Mockingbird* (New York: Harper Perennial, 1960), 18, 21–25.

2. For the purposes of this discussion the term "rural" includes towns and villages, with populations under 2,500 residents, that were not contiguous with cities. This is consistent with the definition adopted by the U.S. Census Bureau.

3. See, for example, Ruth Estella Church, *A Survey of County Public Health Nursing in Wisconsin* (MS thesis, University of Wisconsin, Madison, 1935).

4. *Report of the Committee of Twelve on Rural Schools* (Chicago: National Education Association, 1897), 51.

5. A. C. Monahan, *The Status of Rural Education in the United States* (Washington, DC: U.S. Department of the Interior, Bureau of Education, 1913), 13.

6. Conrad E. Patzer, *Public Education in Wisconsin* (Madison, WI: Department of Public Instruction, 1924), 202–205.

7. I. A. Foster and Harriet Fulmer, *A Health Survey of White County, Illinois* (Springfield: Illinois Board of Health, 1916), 10, 12.
8. Thomas D. Wood, *Minimum Health Requirements for Rural Schools* (Chicago: Press of the American Medical Association, 1920), 9.
9. Katherine Cook, "What Parents Should Know about Their Schools," in *Source Material for the Use of Rural Parent-Teacher Association Units* (Washington, DC: National Congress of Parents and Teachers, 1927), 23.
10. For example, in 1923, only 10 percent of the rural schools in Wyoming had a source of water nearby. *Hot Lunches for Wyoming Rural Schools* (Laramie: Wyoming Extension Service, 1923), 3.
11. David B. Danbom, *Born in the Country: A History of Rural America* (Baltimore: Johns Hopkins University Press, 2006), 161.
12. See, for example, Almeda Brown, *Food Habits of Farm Families* (Logan: Utah Agricultural Experiment Station, 1929); Margaret Coffin, *The Sources of the Food Used by Maryland Farmers* (College Park: Maryland Agricultural Experiment Station, 1933).
13. J. Mace Andress, *Health Education in Rural Schools* (Boston: Houghton Mifflin, 1919), 287–288.
14. Ibid., 287.
15. *Preliminary Report on Conditions and Needs of Rural Schools in Wisconsin* (New York: New York Bureau of Municipal Research, 1912), 34.
16. Nellie Wing Farnsworth, *The Rural School Lunch* (St. Paul, MN: Webb Publishing, 1916), 7.
17. *Historical Statistics of the United States: Colonial Times to 1970* (Washington, DC: U.S. Department of Commerce, Bureau of the Census, 1975), 468.
18. Mary L. Bull, "Hot Lunches in Rural Schools," Fourth International Congress on School Hygiene, Buffalo, NY, 1913, *Transactions*, vol. 5 (Buffalo: Courier, 1914), 320.
19. Farnsworth, *Rural School Lunch*, 7–8; Bull, "Hot Lunches in Rural Schools," 322.
20. Margaret Craig Curran, "Warm Lunches in Country Schools," *Northwest Journal of Education* 23, no. 3 (1911): 168.
21. "School in New Hope Installs Lunch Set," *Stevens Point (WI) Gazette*, 13 December 1922, 5.
22. Eva Robinson Dawes, *The Hot Lunch in the Rural Schools* (Pierre: South Dakota State Department of Public Instruction, 1918), 5–7.
23. Louise Sublette, *I Remember School Lunch: Recollections of Forty-Five Years in School Food Service* (Martin, TN: S&S Book Co., 1976), 169.
24. Julia O. Newton and May C. McDonald, *The Rural Hot Lunch* (Fargo: North Dakota Agricultural College, 1919), 4.
25. Robert L. Leight and Alice Duffy Rinehart, *Country School Memories: An Oral History of One-Room Schooling* (Westport, CT: Greenwood Press, 1999), 100.
26. Waldo L. Adams, "Cafeteria Problems in Rural Schools," *Journal of Home Economics* 24, no. 7 (1932): 598.

27. *Lunches for the Rural School* (Lincoln: University of Nebraska College of Agriculture, 1915), 12.

28. Bull, "Hot Lunches in Rural Schools," 322.

29. Lewis W. Rapeer, *Educational Hygiene from the Pre-School Period to the University* (New York: Charles Scribner's Sons, 1915), 276.

30. Mary Pack, *The School Lunch* (Urbana: University of Illinois College of Agriculture Extension Service, 1921), 10.

31. Anna L. Steckelberg, "Planning for the Hot Lunch in Rural Schools," *Journal of Home Economics* 15, no. 11 (1923): 643.

32. Esther S. Davies, *Food Service in Massachusetts Rural Elementary Schools* (Amherst: Massachusetts Agricultural Experiment Station, 1930), 59.

33. T. A. Erickson, "Hot Lunches for the Country School," *School Education* 31 (1912): 18.

34. W. A. Evans, "How to Keep Well: Warm Lunches at School," *Chicago Daily Tribune*, 31 May 1926, 8.

35. Hamlin Garland, *A Son of the Middle Border* (New York: Grosset & Dunlap, 1917), 115.

36. Farnsworth, *Rural School Lunch*, 6.

37. For example, of the 1,266 men and women enrolled in four Wisconsin normal schools with specific classes on rural teaching, only 97 (7.6 percent) had themselves graduated from high school. In addition, anywhere from one-fourth to one-third of the rural teachers were new each year, as experienced teachers found better-paying positions at graded schools. *Biennial Report of the Department of Public Instruction of the State of Wisconsin, 1908–1910*, 34–35.

38. Steckelberg, "Planning for the Hot Lunch," 646.

39. American Child Health Association, *Report of the Chicago Health Education Conference, 1925* (New York: ACHA, 1926), 221–22.

40. W. W. Trent, *Mountaineer Education: A Story of Education in West Virginia, 1885–1957* (Charleston: Jarrett Printing, 1960), 121.

41. Jerry Apps, *One-Room Country Schools: History and Recollections from Wisconsin* (Amherst, WI: Amherst Press, 1996), 64.

42. *Nutrition and the School Lunch* (Harrisburg: Pennsylvania State Department of Public Instruction, 1935), 35.

43. Price County Nurse, "What Is the Hot Lunch?" (c. 1922), Price County Series, Box 2, "Publicity," no. 78, Wisconsin State Historical Society Archives.

44. Gladys Stillman, *The Hot Lunch in Rural Schools* (Madison: University of Wisconsin College of Agriculture Extension Service, 1920), 3.

45. *Congressional Record*, 78th Congress, 1st Session, 7 April 1943, A1677.

46. Wayne D. Rasmussen and Gladys L. Baker, *The Department of Agriculture* (New York: Praeger, 1972), 243.

47. *Report of the Commissioner of Agriculture* (Washington, DC: U.S. Department of Agriculture, 1888), 13.

48. 28 Stat. L. 271 (8 August 1894), as cited in Paul V. Betters, *The Bureau of Home Economics: Its History, Activities and Organization* (Washington, DC: Brookings Institution, 1930), 83.

49. Norwood Allen Kerr, *The Legacy: A Centennial History of the State Agricultural Experiment Stations, 1887–1987* (Columbia: Missouri Agricultural Experiment Station, 1987), 20.

50. It is impossible to provide substantial empirical evidence to support this claim. Most states kept only minimal records about rural school meal programs, if they kept any at all, and even fewer have survived. Unlike city boards of education, which published detailed annual reports and minutes of meetings, most rural boards disseminated few public records. However, the evidence I have been able to collect suggests that the level of school meal program development in rural Wisconsin was considerably higher than in the rural areas of most, if not all, other states.

51. Only one other state, Vermont, passed such a law before the federal programs that began in the late 1930s rendered such legislation unnecessary. For a more detailed discussion of the legality of school meal programs, see chapter 2.

52. Church, *Survey of County Public Health Nursing in Wisconsin*, 4; Mary V. H. Jones, "The Development of Public Health Nursing in Wisconsin in Relation to Tuberculosis: The Early Years, 1903–1925" (MA thesis, University of Wisconsin, Madison, 1981), 59–60.

53. "Nellie Jones," Biographical File, University Archives, Steenbock Library, University of Wisconsin, Madison; "Nellie Kedzie Jones" (accessed 25 January 2010), available at http://tiny.cc/8l82gy.

54. Grace Langdon, "Hot Lunch in Rural Schools of State: Half of Institutions Banish Cold Food Served to Thousands Each Noon in Past," *Wisconsin State Journal*, 1 January 1922, 30.

55. Gladys Stillman, "Hot Lunches for Rural Schools" (1919), Home Demonstration Agent Reports, Series 9/6/2, Box 48, University Archives, Steenbock Library, University of Wisconsin, Madison.

56. Gladys Stillman, *Annual Report of Child Feeding Specialist* (Madison: University of Wisconsin College of Agriculture Extension Service, 1920), 1–3, Home Demonstration Agent Reports, Series 9/6/2, Box 44, University Archives, Steenbock Library, University of Wisconsin, Madison.

57. "School Inspection Reports, Shawano County, Wisconsin," School Inspection Reports and Records, Shawano Series 12, Box 2, Green Bay Area Research Center, Wisconsin State Historical Society Archives.

58. *Annual Report of the Superintendent of Schools of Shawano County, Wisconsin, 1921–1922*, 2.

59. Langdon, "Hot Lunch in Rural Schools of State," 30; Stillman, *Annual Report of Child Feeding Specialist* (1920), 3; Gladys Stillman, "Hot Lunch for the Rural School," *Child Welfare Magazine* 15, no. 7 (1921): 149.

60. Mary Pack, *The School Lunch* (Urbana: University of Illinois College of Agriculture Extension Service, 1921), 3.

61. Gladys Stillman, *Annual Report of Nutrition Specialist* (Madison: University of Wisconsin College of Agriculture Extension Service, 1921), 4, Home Demonstration Agent Reports, Series 9/6/2, Box 44, University Archives, Steenbock Library, University of Wisconsin, Madison.

62. Gladys Stillman, *Annual Report of Milk Specialist and Assistant Leader* (Madison: University of Wisconsin College of Agriculture Extension Service, 1923), 11, Home Demonstration Agent Reports, Series 9/6/2, Box 44, University Archives, Steenbock Library, University of Wisconsin, Madison.

63. "Health Promotion Week, October 6th to 10th," *Sauk County Schools* 11, no. 1 (1919).

64. According to a survey conducted in 1934 of 12,057 children at 378 schools in twelve Wisconsin counties, 31.1 percent reported drinking coffee daily, and 9.7 percent reported drinking tea daily. See Gladys Stillman, *Milk Drinking Survey of Rural School Children* (Madison: Wisconsin State Department of Public Health, April 1934), Nutrition Division Files, Series 2712, Box 2, Folder 34, Wisconsin State Historical Society Archives.

65. "Something about Coffee," *Sauk County Schools* 11, no. 5 (1920).

66. Letter from the State Superintendent to Laura Jamieson, Portage, WI, 20 February 1922, General Correspondence of the State Superintendent, Series 651, Box 1, Wisconsin State Historical Society Archives.

67. Letter from the State Superintendent to Door County Superintendents Katharine Conley and Thos. Frawley, 9 November 1921, General Correspondence of the State Superintendent, Series 651, Box 1, Wisconsin State Historical Society Archives.

68. Letter from the State Superintendent to Barron County Superintendent August Newman, 9 October 1928, General Correspondence of the State Superintendent, Series 651, Box 3, Wisconsin State Historical Society Archives.

69. Letter from the State Superintendent to Supervising Teachers L. Hanson and E. Jackson, Portage, WI, 29 September 1928, General Correspondence of the State Superintendent, Series 651, Box 3, Wisconsin State Historical Society Archives.

Chapter 5 — "A Nation Ill-Housed, Ill-Clad, Ill-Nourished"

1. Farm incomes and rural purchasing power both increased between 1923 and 1929, but not to prewar levels, and the increases did not offset the precipitous decline in land values and the high start-up costs of mechanized farming. See David E. Hamilton, *From New Day to New Deal: American Farm Policy from Hoover to Roosevelt, 1928–1933* (Chapel Hill: University of North Carolina Press, 1991), 10–11.

2. Paul S. Boyer, ed., *The Oxford Companion to United States History* (New York: Oxford University Press, 2001), 184; Alan Lawson, *A Commonwealth of Hope: The New Deal Response to Crisis* (Baltimore: Johns Hopkins University Press, 2006), 8, 30.

3. Hamilton, *From New Day to New Deal*, 9–11.

4. Janet Poppendieck, *Breadlines Knee-Deep in Wheat: Food Assistance in the Great Depression* (New Brunswick, NJ: Rutgers University Press, 1986), xi.

5. Ibid., 16–17.

6. National School Lunch Act, Pub. L. 396, 79th Congress, 2nd Session (4 June 1946), § 2.

7. David E. Hamilton, "Herbert Hoover and the Great Drought of 1930," *Journal of American History* 68, no. 4 (1982): 850–852, 860. See also Robert Cowley, "The Drought and the Dole: Herbert Hoover's Dismal Dilemma," *American Heritage* 23, no. 2 (1972): 16–19, 92–99; Michele Landis Dauber, *The Sympathetic State: Disaster Relief and the Origins of the American Welfare State* (Chicago: University of Chicago Press, 2013), ch. 4.

8. Poppendieck, *Breadlines Knee-Deep in Wheat*, 30–31.

9. Hamilton, "Herbert Hoover and the Great Drought."

10. Poppendieck, *Breadlines Knee-Deep in Wheat*, 29–31, 35 ff.

11. Ibid., 71.

12. Ibid., 52–53.

13. Ibid., 136.

14. Woody Guthrie, "Plow Under," on *Songs for John Doe* by the Almanac Singers (1941).

15. "Detroit Schools Give Free Lunches," *Pittsburgh Courier*, 13 September 1930, A9.

16. *Annual Report of the Board of Education of the City of St. Louis, Missouri, 1933–1934*, 155.

17. Allen M. Kerr, "Effect of the Economic Crisis on the Nutrition of School Children," *Pennsylvania Medical Journal* 37 (1933): 232–234.

18. George H. Chatfield, *Child Nutrition: 180,000,000 Lunches* (New York: N.p., 1941); "O'Shea Calls Staff to 'War on Hunger,'" *New York Times*, 27 January 1932, 17; "School Relief Fund Faces Wider Need," *New York Times*, 31 January 1932, N2.

19. "Give Lunches Daily to 15,000 in Schools," *New York Times*, 1 April 1932, 14.

20. "Cooperative Extension Work in Agriculture and Home Economics," University of Wisconsin, College of Agriculture (1934), Nutrition Division Files, Series 2712, Box 2, Folder 34, Wisconsin State Historical Society Archives.

21. Blanche M. Stover, "A School Cooperative Cafeteria," *Journal of Home Economics* 25, no. 9 (1933): 759–760. The town of Greenview, Illinois, established a similar program. See Luella A. Williams, "Correlating Class Activities and Community Needs with the School Lunch," *Journal of Home Economics* 25, no. 9 (1933): 756–758.

22. Letter from Ada A. Newman to Lillian A. Lyon, 20 October 1932, District Advisory Nurses' Narrative Reports, 1925–1968, Series 908, Box 1, Folder "Janesville," Wisconsin State Historical Society Archives.

23. C. C. Menzler, *School Lunch Program* (Nashville: Tennessee State Emergency Relief Administration, 1933).

24. Lola Barry, *A Study of the Hot School Lunch in the Rural Schools of Knox County* (MA thesis, University of Tennessee, 1934), 9.

25. *The Emergency Work Relief Program of the F.E.R.A., April 1, 1934–July 1, 1935* (Washington, DC: U.S. Federal Emergency Relief Administration, 1935), 77; H. M. Southworth and M. I. Klayman, *The School Lunch Program and Agricultural Surplus Disposal* (Washington, DC: U.S. Department of Agriculture, 1941), 14–15.

26. The Works Progress Administration was renamed the Work Projects Administration in 1939.

27. *Final Report on the WPA Program, 1935–43* (Washington, DC: U.S. Federal Works Agency, Work Projects Administration, 1946), 68.

28. Ellen S. Woodward, "The Works Progress Administration School Lunch Project," *Journal of Home Economics* 28, no. 9 (1936): 594.

29. Agricultural Adjustment Act, Pub. L. 320, 74th Congress, 2nd Session (24 August 1935), § 32.

30. *Report of the Federal Surplus Commodities Corporation for the Calendar Year 1936* (Washington, DC: U.S. Government Printing Office, 1937), 1.

31. *Report of the Associate Administrator of the Agricultural Adjustment Administration, in Charge of the Division of Marketing and Marketing Agreements, and the President of the Federal Surplus Commodities Corporation, 1939* (Washington, DC: U.S. Government Printing Office), 54.

32. "U.S. Farm Outlets Help Balance Loss," *New York Times*, 29 January 1941, 29.

33. Southworth and Klayman, *School Lunch Program*, 17.

34. Ibid., 30.

35. *Report of the Administrator of the Surplus Marketing Administration, 1941* (Washington, DC: U.S. Government Printing Office, 1942), 20–21.

36. Southworth and Klayman, *School Lunch Program*, 45.

37. Geoffrey S. Shepherd, *Agricultural Price Control* (Ames: Iowa State College Press, 1945), 175.

38. William Gammon, *U.S. Civil Works Administration of Missouri: A Review, November 15, 1933, to March 31, 1934* (Jefferson City: Missouri State Relief and Reconstruction Commission, 1934), table XI.

39. Hazel K. Stiebeling, *Are We Well Fed? A Report on the Diets of Families in the United States* (Washington, DC: U.S. Department of Agriculture, Bureau of Home Economics, 1941), 3, 7.

40. See, for example, Alberta B. Childs, "Some Dietary Studies of Poles, Mexicans, Italians, and Negroes," *Child Health Bulletin* 9 (1933): 84–91; Mary E. Frayser and Ada M. Moser, *The Diet of School Children in Relation to Their Health* (Clemson: South Carolina Agricultural Experiment Station, Clemson Agricultural College, 1930); Jet C. Winters, "A Study of the Diet of Mexicans Living in Texas," *Journal of the American Dietetic Association* 8, no. 1 (1932): 47–55.

41. During World War II, medical examiners rejected 45 percent of the 2.7 million men who were examined, a considerably higher rejection rate than that of World War I. Direct comparison of the two cases is virtually impossible; some of the differences between the rejection statistics of the two wars can be attributed to changes in military benchmarks, diagnostic standards, and examination techniques, both comprehensive and individual. Furthermore, during World War II, physicians examined only those men with no dependents or other reason for deferment; they had examined all men seeking deferment during World War I. However, as the chief of the Division of Public Health Methods of the USPHS noted, "there is certainly no evidence of any improvement in the physical status of young men since World War I" (G. St. J. Perrott, "Findings of Selective Service Examinations," *Milbank Memorial Fund Quarterly* 22 [1944]: 358). Between the wars, the national mortality rate dropped by over three per thousand despite the hardships of the Great Depression, but morbidity rates seemed to be increasing. According to Surgeon General Thomas Parran, "undoubtedly a large amount of ill health and a large amount of rejections under Selective Service have a nutritional base" (*Bills Relating to the School Lunch Program: Hearings before the Committee on Agriculture, United States House of Representatives, 79th Congress, 1st Session, on H.R. 2673, H.R. 3143 [H.R. 3370 Reported]* [1945], 22; see also *Congressional Record*, 78th Congress, 2nd Session, 2 May 1944, 3845). Indeed, children with low weights were more likely to be rejected by draft boards as adults than children with normal weights, suggesting significant long-term consequences for even moderate malnourishment (Antonio Ciocco, Henry Klein, and Carroll E. Palmer, "Child Health and the Selective Service Physical Standards," *Public Health Reports* 56, no. 50 [1941]: 2372).
42. Pearl A. Wanamaker, *State of Washington Community School Lunch Program* (Olympia: State Superintendent of Public Instruction, 1942), 5. See also *Hunger Quits School* (Washington, DC: U.S. Department of Agriculture, Food Distribution Administration, 1943), 8.
43. Ada M. Moser, *School Lunches in Two Rural Communities* (Clemson: South Carolina Agricultural Experiment Station, Clemson Agricultural College, 1943), 10.
44. *School Lunch and Milk Programs: Hearings before a Subcommittee of the Committee on Agriculture and Forestry, United States Senate, 78th Congress, 2nd Session, on S. 1820 and S. 1824* (1944), 57.
45. Shepherd, *Agricultural Price Control*, 150.
46. Southworth and Klayman, *School Lunch Program*, 27–28.
47. Ibid., 26, 48–49.
48. Ibid., 20, 22.
49. *School Lunch and Milk Programs*, 14.
50. Marjorie M. Heseltine, "The Nutritionist in Public Health Work," *Journal of the American Dietetic Association* 14, no. 4 (1938): 243;

Martha M. Eliot and Marjorie M. Heseltine, "Nutrition in Maternal and Child Health Programs," *Nutrition Reviews* 5, no. 2 (1947): 34. See also E. V. McCollum, "Report of Round-Table on Nutrition and Public Health," in *New Health Frontiers: Proceedings of the 15th Annual Conference of the Milbank Memorial Fund* (New York: Milbank Memorial Fund, 1937), 61–75.

51. *Bills Relating to the School Lunch Program*, 110, 113, 243.

52. *School Lunch and Milk Programs*, 84.

53. Ibid., 117.

54. *Bills Relating to the School Lunch Program*, 109.

55. A. R. Ruis, "'Children with Half-Starved Bodies' and the Assessment of Malnutrition in the United States, 1890–1950," *Bulletin of the History of Medicine* 87, no. 3 (2013): 380–408.

56. *School Lunch and Milk Programs*, 159.

57. James A. Wilson, *The Place of the Community Gardens in the School Lunch Program with Special Reference to Utilization of Agricultural Surpluses in Correcting Prevalent Child Malnutrition* (Sacramento: California State Relief Administration, 1940), 2.

58. *Report on Progress of the WPA Program, June 30, 1942* (Washington, DC: U.S. Government Printing Office), 48–49.

59. Bena Johnson, "School Lunches Carry on in Minnesota," *Journal of Home Economics* 35, no. 5 (1943): 279.

60. Wilson, *Place of the Community Gardens in the School Lunch Program*, 1. For discussion of a locally organized garden program, see Kathleen R. Babbitt, "Legitimizing Nutrition Education: The Impact of The Great Depression," in *Rethinking Home Economics: Women and the History of a Profession*, ed. Sarah Stage and Virginia B. Vincenti (Ithaca, NY: Cornell University Press, 1997), 159 ff.

61. *Annual Report of the Board of Directors of the School District of Kansas City, Missouri, 1912–13*, 121.

62. *School Gardens for School Lunches* (Washington, DC: U.S. Office of Education, Federal Security Agency, 1942), 3.

63. Southworth and Klayman, *School Lunch Program*, 30.

64. Edwin B. Angier, "Your 'Food for Freedom' Garden," *Los Angeles School Journal* 25, no. 21 (1942): 10–11; *Gardening through the Schools* (Sacramento: California State Department of Education, 1942); Clayton F. Palmer, "Children and Victory Gardens," *Los Angeles School Journal* 25, no. 21 (1942): 8–9. On the broader ways in which World War II affected eating, see Amy Bentley, *Eating for Victory: Food Rationing and the Politics of Domesticity* (Urbana: University of Illinois Press, 1998).

65. *Congressional Record*, 78th Congress, 2nd Session, 1 June 1944, 5168.

66. *Congressional Record*, 79th Congress, 2nd Session, 19 February 1946, 1466.

67. Southworth and Klayman, *School Lunch Program*, 30.

Chapter 6 — From Aid to Entitlement

1. Rowena S. Carpenter and Margaret Marco Morris, "Wartime Aid to School Lunches," *Journal of Home Economics* 35, no. 9 (1943): 553–554; *The Community School Lunch Program* (Washington, DC: U.S. War Food Administration, Office of Distribution, 1944), 4.
2. Ethel Austin Martin, "Building a Health Program around the School Lunch," *Practical Home Economics* 8 (1930): 38.
3. *School Lunch and Milk Programs: Hearings before a Subcommittee of the Committee on Agriculture and Forestry, United States Senate, 78th Congress, 2nd Session, on S. 1820 and S. 1824* (2 May 1944), 116.
4. H. M. Southworth and M. I. Klayman, *The School Lunch Program and Agricultural Surplus Disposal* (Washington, DC: U.S. Department of Agriculture, 1941), 36–37.
5. *Final Report on the WPA Program, 1935–43* (Washington, DC: U.S. Government Printing Office, 1946), 36.
6. *School Lunch and Milk Programs*, 30.
7. Thomas A. Becnel, *Senator Allen Ellender of Louisiana: A Biography* (Baton Rouge: Louisiana State University Press, 1995), 78 ff.; Gilbert C. Fite, *Richard B. Russell, Jr., Senator from Georgia* (Chapel Hill: University of North Carolina Press, 1991), 186–189.
8. *School Lunch and Milk Programs*, 17.
9. Ibid., 35.
10. Ibid., 43.
11. Ibid., 70, 90.
12. Ibid., 241.
13. Ibid., 59.
14. *Congressional Record*, 78th Congress, 2nd Session, 17 April 1944, A1818. On Thompson and her influence, see "Cartwheel Girl," *Time*, 12 June 1939, 27.
15. *Congressional Record*, 79th Congress, 2nd Session, 19 February 1946, 1455–1456.
16. Ibid., 1456.
17. Ibid., 1451 ff.
18. *Bills Relating to the School Lunch Program: Hearings before the Committee on Agriculture, United States House of Representatives, 79th Congress, 1st Session, on H.R. 2673, H.R. 3143 (H.R. 3370 Reported)* (Washington, DC, 1945), 14, 25 ff., 34 ff.
19. *Congressional Record*, 79th Congress, 2nd Session, 19 February 1946, 1475.
20. *Congressional Record*, 78th Congress, 2nd Session, 1 June 1944, 5164.
21. Ibid., 5162, 5169.
22. *Congressional Record*, 78th Congress, 2nd Session, 2 May 1944, 3845 ff.
23. *Congressional Record*, 78th Congress, 1st Session, 11 June 1943, 5703–5704.

24. *Congressional Record*, 78th Congress, 2nd Session, 1 June 1944, 5165.

25. *Congressional Record*, 79th Congress, 2nd Session, 18 February 1946, 1382.

26. *Congressional Record*, 79th Congress, 1st Session, 24 March 1945, 2721.

27. Ibid., 2724.

28. *Bills Relating to the School Lunch Program*, 53.

29. Ibid., 2.

30. *Congressional Record*, 79th Congress, 1st Session, 24 March 1945, 2722–2723; cf. ibid., 2725.

31. *Congressional Record*, 79th Congress, 2nd Session, 12 February 1946, A890.

32. *Congressional Record*, 79th Congress, 2nd Session, 26 February 1946, 1611.

33. *Congressional Record*, 79th Congress, 2nd Session, 19 February 1946, 1454, 1469.

34. *Congressional Record*, 79th Congress, 2nd Session, 26 February 1946, 1611.

35. *Congressional Record*, 79th Congress, 2nd Session, 19 Feburary 1946, 1477.

36. John Flannagan, *School Lunch Program: Report to Accompany H.R. 3370*, H.R. Report No. 684, 79th Congress, 1st Session (5 June 1945).

37. Allen Ellender, *Providing Assistance to the States in the Establishment, Maintenance, Operation, and Expansion of School-Lunch Programs: Report to Accompany S. 962*, S. Report No. 553, 79th Congress, 1st Session (28 July 1945), 16.

38. *School Lunch and Milk Programs*, 23. See also *Bills Relating to the School Lunch Program*, 2.

39. *Congressional Record*, 79th Congress, 2nd Session, 15 February 1946, A779.

40. *Congressional Record*, 79th Congress, 1st Session, 8 February 1945, 924.

41. *Congressional Record*, 79th Congress, 2nd Session, 19 February 1946, 1460.

42. Ibid.

43. *Congressional Record*, 79th Congress, 2nd Session, 21 February 1946, 1537.

44. Ibid., 1534 ff.

45. *Congressional Record*, 79th Congress, 2nd Session, 26 February 1946, 1626–1628. On the conservative coalition, see James T. Patterson, "A Conservative Coalition Forms in Congress, 1933–1939," *Journal of American History* 52, no. 4 (1966): 757–772.

46. Mark V. Tushnet, *The NAACP's Legal Strategy against Segregated Education, 1925–1950* (Chapel Hill: University of North Carolina Press, 1987), 5–6.

47. Harvard Sitkoff, *A New Deal for Blacks: The Emergence of Civil Rights as a National Issue* (New York: Oxford University Press, 1978), 35–36, 48–49.

48. *Historical Statistics of the United States: Colonial Times to the Present* (Washington, DC: U.S. Department of Commerce, Bureau of the Census, 1960), 25; Forrest E. Linder and Robert D. Grove, *Vital Statistics Rates in the United States, 1900–1940* (Washington, DC: 1947), 122–124. On the history of black health in the early twentieth century, see Vanessa Northington Gamble, *Making a Place for Ourselves: The Black Hospital Movement, 1920–1945* (New York: Oxford University Press, 1995); James H. Jones, *Bad Blood: The Tuskegee Syphilis Experiment* (New York: Free Press, 1993); David McBride, *From TB to AIDS: Epidemics among Urban Blacks since 1900* (Albany: State University of New York Press, 1991); Susan M. Reverby, ed., *Tuskegee's Truths: Rethinking the Tuskegee Syphilis Study* (Chapel Hill: University of North Carolina Press, 2000); Samuel Kelton Roberts Jr., *Infectious Fear: Politics, Disease, and the Health Effects of Segregation* (Chapel Hill: University of North Carolina Press, 2009); Susan L. Smith, *Sick and Tired of Being Sick and Tired: Black Women's Health Activism in America, 1890–1950* (Philadelphia: University of Pennsylvania Press, 1995); Keith Wailoo, *Dying in the City of the Blues: Sickle Cell Anemia and the Politics of Race and Health* (Chapel Hill: University of North Carolina Press, 2001).

49. *Congressional Record*, 79th Congress, 2nd Session, 20 February 1946, 1493.

50. Ellender, *Providing Assistance to the States*, 17.

51. *Congressional Record*, 79th Congress, 2nd Session, 19 February 1946, 1456.

52. *Congressional Record*, 79th Congress, 2nd Session, 20 February 1946, 1494.

53. Ellen S. Woodward, "The Works Progress Administration School Lunch Project," *Journal of Home Economics* 28, no. 9 (1936): 594.

54. *Congressional Record*, 79th Congress, 2nd Session, 20 February 1946, 1495.

55. *Congressional Record*, 78th Congress, 2nd Session, 19 May 1944, A2458.

56. *Congressional Record*, 79th Congress, 2nd Session, 19 February 1946, 1453.

57. Ibid., 1477.

58. Ibid., 1478.

59. *Bills Relating to the School Lunch Program*, 29.

60. The House members of the joint committee were August Andresen, Harold Cooley, John Flannagan, Clifford Hope, Stephen Pace, and Orville Zimmerman; the Senate members were George Aiken, John Bankhead, Arthur Capper, Allen Ellender, and Richard Russell.

61. John Flannagan, *School-Lunch Program: Report to Accompany H.R. 3370*, H.R. Report No. 2080, 79th Congress, 2nd Session (20 May 1946), 2–4.

62. Ibid., 5.

63. *Congressional Record*, 79th Congress, 2nd Session, 7 March 1946, A1192.

64. Flannagan, *School-Lunch Program* (1946), 1.

65. Ibid., 4.

66. National School Lunch Act, Pub. L. 396, 79th Congress, 2nd Session (4 June 1946).

67. Ibid., § 9.

68. Ibid., § 7.

69. Susan Levine, *School Lunch Politics: The Surprising History of America's Favorite Welfare Program* (Princeton: Princeton University Press, 2008), ch. 4.

70. *Congressional Record*, 79th Congress, 2nd Session, 27 February 1946, 1697–98.

71. *Congressional Record*, 79th Congress, 2nd Session, 19 February 1946, 1455.

72. For discussions of the NSLP, see Levine, *School Lunch Politics*; Janet Poppendieck, *Free for All: Fixing School Food in America* (Berkeley: University of California Press, 2010); Norwood Allen Kerr, "Drafted into the War on Poverty: USDA Food and Nutrition Programs, 1961–1969," *Agricultural History* 64, no. 2 (1990): 154–166; J. Amy Dillard, "Sloppy Joe, Slop, Sloppy Joe: How USDA Commodities Dumping Ruined the National School Lunch Program," *Oregon Law Review* 87, no. 1 (2008): 221–257; Jennifer E. Gaddis, "Mobilizing to Re-value and Re-skill Foodservice Labor in US School Lunchrooms: A Pathway to Community-Level Food Sovereignty?" *Radical Teacher* 98 (2014): 15–21; Nicholas Confessore, "How School Lunch Became the Latest Political Battleground," *New York Times Magazine*, 7 October 2014, 34–40, 86, 93–94.

73. *National School Lunch Act*, § 11c.

74. Annelise Orleck, *Storming Caesars Palace: How Black Mothers Fought Their Own War on Poverty* (Boston: Beacon Press, 2005), 176–177.

Epilogue

1. Charles Douglas, "The Laws of Nutrition Should Be Taught in the Schools," *Physician and Surgeon* 21, no. 11 (1899): 495–496.

2. *Bills Relating to the School Lunch Program: Hearings before the Committee on Agriculture, United States House of Representatives, 79th Congress, 1st Session, on H.R. 2673, H.R. 3143 (H.R. 3370 Reported)* (1945), 14.

3. Timothy Egan, "In Bid to Improve Nutrition, Schools Expel Soda and Chips," *New York Times*, 20 May 2002, A1; "High School Lunch Room: Pupils to Be Hygienically Fed at Low Prices," *New Haven Evening Register*, 8 November 1897, 1.

4. *The Surgeon General's Call to Action to Prevent and Decrease Overweight and Obesity* (Rockville, MD: U.S. Department of Health and Human Services, Office of the Surgeon General, 2001), xiii.

5. *School Lunches and Education: Helps from Federal Agencies* (Washington, DC: U.S. Office of Education, 1942), 4.

6. Roland Sturm and Kenneth B. Wells, *The Health Risks of Obesity: Worse than Smoking, Drinking, or Poverty* (Santa Monica, CA: RAND Corporation, 2002).

7. Michael Pollan, *The Omnivore's Dilemma: A Natural History of Four Meals* (New York: Penguin, 2006); Eric Schlosser, *Fast Food Nation: The Dark Side of the All-American Meal* (New York: Harper Perennial, 2001); Morgan Spurlock, *Super Size Me* (documentary film, 2004); Robert Hunter, *Poverty: Social Conscience in the Progressive Era* (New York: Macmillan, 1904); Upton Sinclair, *The Jungle* (New York: Doubleday, Jabber, 1906); John Spargo, *Underfed School Children: The Problem and the Remedy* (Chicago: Charles H. Kerr, 1906).

8. See, for example, William Christeson, Amy Dawson Taggart, and Soren Messner-Zidell, *Too Fat to Fight* (Washington, DC: Mission: Readiness, 2010), 3.

9. Egan, "In Bid to Improve Nutrition," A1, A16.

10. Virginia A. Stallings, Carol West Suitor, and Christine L. Taylor, *School Meals: Building Blocks for Healthy Children* (Washington, DC: Institute of Medicine, Food and Nutrition Board, 2010).

11. *The School Health Program: Report of the Committee on the School Child, White House Conference on Child Health and Protection, Section III: Education and Training* (New York: Century, 1932), 123.

12. Egan, "In Bid to Improve Nutrition," A16.

13. Anonymous elementary school principals quoted in Lydia J. Roberts, *Nutrition Work with Children* (Chicago: University of Chicago Press, 1927), 261.

14. Kim Severson, "School's Toughest Test: Cooking," *New York Times*, 30 September 2009.

15. Heather Graham and Sheri Zidenberg-Cherr, "California Teachers Perceive School Gardens as an Effective Nutritional Tool to Promote Healthful Eating Habits," *Journal of the American Dietetic Association* 105, no. 11 (2005): 1797–1800; Jennifer L. Morris and Sheri Zidenberg-Cherr, "Garden-Enhanced Nutrition Curriculum Improves Fourth-Grade School Children's Knowledge of Nutrition and Preferences for Some Vegetables," *Journal of the American Dietetic Association* 102, no. 1 (2002): 91–93.

16. Katharine Mieszkowski, "School Cafeteria's Fruits and Vegetables Vie with Food Trucks' Sweet and Salty Treats," *New York Times*, 10 September 2011.

17. Healthy, Hunger-Free Kids Act, Pub. L. 111–296, 111th Congress, 2nd Session (13 December 2010), §§ 204, 208.

18. Jennifer E. Gaddis, "Mobilizing to Re-value and Re-skill Foodservice Labor in U.S. School Lunchrooms: A Pathway to Community-Level Food Sovereignty?" *Radical Teacher* 98 (2014): 15–21.

Index

academic achievement, 12, 18, 65, 133, 147

adulteration. *See* food, safety of

Agricultural Adjustment Act, 118–119, 123, 139

Agricultural Adjustment Administration, 118–119

agricultural economics, 9, 111–112, 114, 119, 121

agricultural experiment stations, 97, 102, 127

AICP. *See* New York Association for Improving the Condition of the Poor

American Dietetic Association, 139, 156

American Medical Association, 11

American Red Cross, 101, 116–117

Baker, S. Josephine, 17, 76–77

breakfast, 27, 33, 59, 81, 92. *See also* school breakfast

canning, 130–132

central kitchen, 22, 70, 73, 76

Chatfield, George, 65, 67, 129–130

Chicago School Extension Committee (CSEC), 38–43, 47

coffee, 27–29, 54, 69, 84, 98, 108, 180n22

compulsory education, 6, 11, 14, 63

concessionaires, 40, 60, 79–80, 83–84

cooperative cafeterias, 121, 163

diet, 29, 56–57, 59, 68–69, 71–72, 83–84, 91, 127–128, 130, 160

dietitians. *See* nutritionists

digestion, 99–100, 102

Dilweg, La Vern, 152, 154

disaster relief, 116–118

Ellender, Allen, 138–140, 146–147, 151

Emerson, Haven, 74, 78–79

expertise, 129, 152

Extension Service, 9, 17, 101–103, 104–105, 107, 110, 123, 129

farm-to-school programs, 121, 161–164

Federal Emergency Relief Association, 122

Federal Farm Board, 117, 118

Federal Surplus Commodities Corporation, 124–125, 129

Federal Surplus Relief Corporation, 119, 124

fireless cooker, 97

Flannagan, John, 141, 142, 145, 146, 150, 154

food: and assistance programs, 117, 155; distribution of, 73–74, 119, 122–126, 128, 132, 135–136, 164; junk, 2, 28–29, 53–56, 70, 84, 160–161, 163; processed, 3, 130, 162; safety of, 29–30, 43, 60, 70–71, 74, 84; surpluses of, 3, 10, 113–120, 123–132, 135, 138–140, 142–146, 154, 160–164

food carts, 23, 27–30, 62, 66, 69–71, 75

food security, 2, 9, 20, 112, 115, 154, 159

Hatch Experiment Station Act, 102–103

Healthy, Hunger-Free Kids Act, 2–3, 163–165

hookworm, 87–88, 91, 101

Hoover, Herbert, 116, 118

hot lunch, 4, 53, 92, 95–100, 104–108, 121, 145, 156–157. *See also* school lunch

About the Author

A. R. Ruis is a historian of medicine and public health and an education researcher at the University of Wisconsin–Madison.

Available titles in the Critical Issues in Health and Medicine series:

Emily K. Abel, *Suffering in the Land of Sunshine: A Los Angeles Illness Narrative*

Emily K. Abel, *Tuberculosis and the Politics of Exclusion: A History of Public Health and Migration to Los Angeles*

Marilyn Aguirre-Molina, Luisa N. Borrell, and William Vega, eds. *Health Issues in Latino Males: A Social and Structural Approach*

Anne-Emanuelle Birn and Theodore M. Brown, eds., Comrades in Health: U.S. Health Internationalists, Abroad and at Home

Susan M. Chambré, *Fighting for Our Lives: New York's AIDS Community and the Politics of Disease*

James Colgrove, Gerald Markowitz, and David Rosner, eds., *The Contested Boundaries of American Public Health*

Cynthia A. Connolly, *Saving Sickly Children: The Tuberculosis Preventorium in American Life, 1909–1970*

Patricia D'Antonio, Nursing with a Message: Public Health Demonstration Projects in New York City

Tasha N. Dubriwny, *The Vulnerable Empowered Woman: Feminism, Postfeminism, and Women's Health*

Edward J. Eckenfels, *Doctors Serving People: Restoring Humanism to Medicine through Student Community Service*

Julie Fairman, *Making Room in the Clinic: Nurse Practitioners and the Evolution of Modern Health Care*

Jill A. Fisher, *Medical Research for Hire: The Political Economy of Pharmaceutical Clinical Trials*

Charlene Galarneau, Communities of Health Care Justice

Alyshia Gálvez, *Patient Citizens, Immigrant Mothers: Mexican Women, Public Prenatal Care and the Birth Weight Paradox*

Gerald N. Grob and Howard H. Goldman, *The Dilemma of Federal Mental Health Policy: Radical Reform or Incremental Change?*

Gerald N. Grob and Allan V. Horwitz, *Diagnosis, Therapy, and Evidence: Conundrums in Modern American Medicine*

Rachel Grob, *Testing Baby: The Transformation of Newborn Screening, Parenting, and Policymaking*

Mark A. Hall and Sara Rosenbaum, eds., *The Health Care "Safety Net" in a Post-Reform World*

Laura L. Heinemann, Transplanting Care: Shifting Commitments in Health and Care in the United States

Laura D. Hirshbein, *American Melancholy: Constructions of Depression in the Twentieth Century*

Laura D. Hirshbein, Smoking Privileges: Psychiatry, the Mentally Ill, and the Tobacco Industry in America

Timothy Hoff, *Practice under Pressure: Primary Care Physicians and Their Medicine in the Twenty-first Century*

Beatrix Hoffman, Nancy Tomes, Rachel N. Grob, and Mark Schlesinger, eds., *Patients as Policy Actors*

Ruth Horowitz, *Deciding the Public Interest: Medical Licensing and Discipline*

Powel Kazanjian, *Frederick Novy and the Development of Bacteriology in American Medicine*

Rebecca M. Kluchin, *Fit to Be Tied: Sterilization and Reproductive Rights in America, 1950–1980*

Jennifer Lisa Koslow, *Cultivating Health: Los Angeles Women and Public Health Reform*

Susan C. Lawrence, Privacy and the Past: Research, Law, Archives, Ethics

Bonnie Lefkowitz, *Community Health Centers: A Movement and the People Who Made It Happen*

Ellen Leopold, *Under the Radar: Cancer and the Cold War*

Barbara L. Ley, *From Pink to Green: Disease Prevention and the Environmental Breast Cancer Movement*

Sonja Mackenzie, *Structural Intimacies: Sexual Stories in the Black AIDS Epidemic*

Michelle McClellan, *Lady Lushes: Gender, Alcohol, and Medicine in Modern America*

David Mechanic, *The Truth about Health Care: Why Reform Is Not Working in America*

Richard A. Meckel, Classrooms and Clinics: Urban Schools and the Protection and Promotion of Child Health, 1870–1930

Alyssa Picard, *Making the American Mouth: Dentists and Public Health in the Twentieth Century*

Heather Munro Prescott, *The Morning After: A History of Emergency Contraception in the United States*

A. R. Ruis, *Eating to Learn, Learning to Eat: The Origins of School Lunch in the United States*

James A. Schafer Jr., The Business of Private Medical Practice: Doctors, Specialization, and Urban Change in Philadelphia, 1900–1940

David G. Schuster, *Neurasthenic Nation: America's Search for Health, Happiness, and Comfort, 1869–1920*

Karen Seccombe and Kim A. Hoffman, *Just Don't Get Sick: Access to Health Care in the Aftermath of Welfare Reform*

Leo B. Slater, *War and Disease: Biomedical Research on Malaria in the Twentieth Century*

Paige Hall Smith, Bernice L. Hausman, and Miriam Labbok, *Beyond Health, Beyond Choice: Breastfeeding Constraints and Realities*

Matthew Smith, *An Alternative History of Hyperactivity: Food Additives and the Feingold Diet*

Susan L. Smith, Toxic Exposures: Mustard Gas and the Health Consequences of World War II in the United States

Rosemary A. Stevens, Charles E. Rosenberg, and Lawton R. Burns, eds., *History and Health Policy in the United States: Putting the Past Back In*

Barbra Mann Wall, *American Catholic Hospitals: A Century of Changing Markets and Missions*

Frances Ward, *The Door of Last Resort: Memoirs of a Nurse Practitioner*

Printed and bound by CPI Group (UK) Ltd, Croydon, CR0 4YY

27/10/2024

14580231-0002

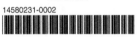